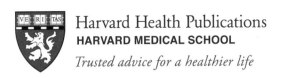

Harvard Health Publications
HARVARD MEDICAL SCHOOL

Trusted advice for a healthier life

Dear Reader,

Every year, at least one out of three people over the age of 65 falls. When a toddler tumbles, he or she may shed a few tears before surging ahead again unscathed. When an adult falls, particularly an older adult, consequences are often far worse. Every year, falls prove fatal for nearly 22,000 people ages 55 or older. But even nonfatal falls can be devastating. Hip fractures and head injuries from falls undermine independence and raise the risk for an early death.

Poor balance, a persistent problem for millions of Americans, triggers many falls. In young, healthy adults, balance is largely an automatic reflex. However, gradual changes linked to growing older—such as weak or inflexible muscles, slower reflexes, and worsening eyesight—affect the sense of balance. Certain health problems—such as inner ear disorders, neuropathy, and heart rhythm disturbances—may upset balance, too. So can alcohol and many medications.

Shaky balance can spur a downward spiral. Often, people begin moving around less during the day, voluntarily cutting back activities. Confidence dips, muscles essential to balance grow weaker still, and unsteadiness rises in response. So does fear of falling—which in turn further constrains a person's activities.

For this report, we've combined our expertise to select safe, effective balance exercises that can help stop this cycle. With practice, almost anyone can achieve better balance. Strong legs and flexible ankles help prevent falls and allow you to catch yourself if you do trip. What's more, the full blend of recommended activities can help you build better awareness of your body and surroundings, boost your confidence, and tune up your heart and lungs to keep you healthy and independent.

Falls occur for many reasons, of course—not just balance problems. Clutter, broken pavement, dim lighting, and even essential medications can play a role. That's why we've included an in-depth section on fall prevention. Our checklists offer step-by-step strategies for fall-proofing yourself and your home.

So, flip through the pages of this Special Health Report. Read the safety and fall-prevention tips. Talk to your doctor about health problems and medications that could play a role in falls. Then get started on the walking plan and balance workouts. Fewer injuries and a restored zest in life are well worth the effort.

Sincerely,

Suzanne Salamon, M.D.
Medical Editor

Brad Manor, Ph.D.
Medical Editor

Josie Gardiner
Master Trainer

Joy Prouty
Master Trainer

Harvard Health Publications | Harvard Medical School | 10 Shattuck Street, Second Floor | Boston, MA 02115

How balance works

Why spend precious time improving your balance? What is balance, anyway, and which systems in the body govern it? This chapter addresses these questions.

Why improve your balance?

Every year, one in three adults 65 or older falls at least once. Over the past decade, deaths from falls have risen sharply for this age group. Of course, most falls are not fatal. However, according to the Centers for Disease Control and Prevention, falls cause 2.3 million nonfatal injuries among older adults every year that are serious enough to merit a trip to the emergency room. Of these accidents, 20% to 30% involved cuts, hip fractures (broken hip bones), or head injuries, undermining independence and raising the risk for early death.

At any age, poor balance can cause falls. A whopping eight million Americans report persistent balance problems, according to the National Institutes of Health. Millions more suffer from chronic dizziness, which also makes people unsteady on their feet.

The body systems responsible for balance can be affected by health problems, medications, or gradual changes that accompany aging. Curtailing activity because of unsteadiness further weakens muscles and erodes balance in a downward spiral. As balance becomes increasingly impaired, simple acts, such as strolling through a grocery store or reaching overhead, become trickier. Stumbles occur more often. Fear of falling ticks upward and confidence declines, virtually imprisoning some people at home.

Good balance, by contrast, helps prevent potentially disabling falls. It builds confidence and fosters independence. If you love tennis, golf, running, dancing, skiing, or any number of other sports or activities, working on balance buffs your abilities. Not an athlete? Just walking across the floor or down the block requires good balance. So does rising from a chair, going up and down stairs, toting packages, and even turning to look behind you.

The balance exercises in this report will make you steadier, more confident, and less likely to fall. We designed progressive challenges, starting with a workout of safe, easy exercises that shouldn't be out of reach for unsteady people of any age. Practicing regularly will ensure that your balance doesn't worsen. Better still, it can help you improve your balance significantly.

Before launching into the workouts, though, it helps to understand how your sense of balance works and how aging, health issues, and various medicines affect it.

The body's balance systems

Balance can be described as the ability to distribute your weight in a way that enables you to hold a steady position or move at will without falling. Static balance helps you stay upright when standing still. Dynamic balance allows you to anticipate and react to changes as you move. Both types of balance work to keep your center of gravity—the point at which body weight is evenly distributed—poised over your base of support.

Our daily balancing acts require interplay among several systems: the central nervous system (brain and spinal cord), the vestibular system (brain and inner ear), the visual system (brain and eye), and a vast web of position-sensing nerves called proprioceptors in far-flung areas of the body. Muscles and bones are pressed into service as well, to turn spinal reflexes and the brain's commands into movement.

Brain. Together, the brain and spinal cord form the central nervous system. The cerebellum, a portion of the brain perched behind the brainstem and below the cerebral cortex, oversees balance and movement. It receives information gathered by a network of sensory nerves and issues commands. It also retrieves stored memories of movements deeply ingrained through practice—for example, walking, riding a bike, or kicking a soccer ball. The cerebral cortex chimes in, too. Home to the frontal lobe, which plays roles in attention, planning, and movement, it supplies other memories important to balance, such as recalled patterns of movement to surmount challenges like a slippery sidewalk or rocky path.

Spinal cord. Housed safely in a channel carved through the vertebrae, the spinal cord serves as a bridge between brain and body. Paired nerves peppered along its length receive feedback from the peripheral nervous system, a lacework of nerve fibers branching out from the central nervous system to the hinterlands of the body. The spinal cord also gives rise to a host of reflexes, such as the quick-stepping response to an unexpected push. It delivers voluntary movement commands to the muscles, too.

Vestibular system. Central to the sense of balance is the vestibular system of the inner ear. It contains several important structures. The labyrinth is a maze of bone and tissue. One end of it houses the cochlea, a spiral-shaped organ essential to hearing. Three semicircular canals, fluid-filled loops set at different angles, lie at the other end. At the base of each loop, a bell-shaped cupula sits above a clump of sensory hair cells, which tilt as thick fluid (endolymph) in the semicircular canal moves. Signals set off by this tilting action travel to the brain via the acoustic nerve, describing the position and rotational movements of your head: straight up and down, side to side, tilting toward one shoulder, and so forth.

Just beyond the semicircular canals are the utricle and the saccule. Dubbed the otolithic organs, these two fluid-filled pouches are also lined with sensory hair cells that inform the brain about head position when you're sitting up, leaning back, or lying down. Inside the pouches, grains of calcium carbonate (canaliths, or otoconia) are sprinkled on top of a layer of gel overlying the hair cells. Each time your head tilts, gravity pulls on these tiny stones. Hair cells shift in response, sending signals to the brain describing the position of your head. The sensory cells in the utricle also report horizontal body movement to the brain—say, when you're walking forward or riding a bike. Those in the saccule monitor vertical acceleration of the body, which would occur if you stood up or rode in an elevator, for example.

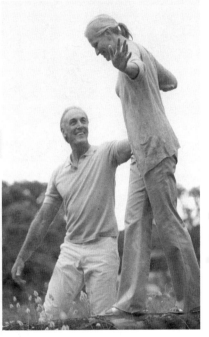

Visual system. The eyes send visual information via the optic nerve to the brain, constantly logging where you are in relation to surrounding objects. Thus, sight is a key supplement to other sensory input and is important to proprioception, the sense of where your body is in relation to its surroundings. If you doubt this, stand next to a counter and lift one of your feet. Now try closing your eyes while lifting your foot. Odds are good that you'll sway more and need to grab on to the counter to steady yourself.

Proprioceptors. These position-sensing nerves are responsible for proprioception, the ability to perceive

Run the numbers

- One out of five fall deaths are in people under 65; four out of five are in people 65 and older.

- Men are more likely to die from falls. Women are more likely to be injured. As one example, older women have more than double the rate of fall-related fractures (broken bones) than men.

- Practically all hip fractures—over 90%—result from falls. Fractures of the spine, forearm, leg, ankle, pelvis, upper arm, and hand are common, too. Of course, the bones that break may already be weakened and brittle because of osteoporosis.

- As many as one in four older adults who lived independently before a hip fracture spends at least a year afterward in a nursing home.

- Complications following a hip fracture or surgery to treat it, such as pneumonia or blood clots, are sometimes fatal.

where your body is in space. Proprioception helps you stay balanced and move through your environment without stumbling or bumping into things. Found primarily in muscles, tendons, and joints, proprioceptors stream information to the brain. The brain then relays commands back down the chain, instructing muscles to adjust contractions in large or small ways as conditions change—when, for example, you stand on an unsteady surface or step off a curb into the street. Proprioceptors in your feet play an especially big role in balance. As you shift from standing to walking forward, for example, pressure rolls toward the front portion of your foot, an act captured by proprioceptors threaded along the sole of the foot and throughout the ankle joint.

Muscles, tendons, and bones. Stretchy cords of tissue called tendons tether muscles to bones and cartilage, the tissue that cushions intersections between bones. Sensory information gathered by proprioceptors is ferried toward the brain via lightning-quick signals sent along nerve pathways. Commands from the brain returned just as speedily prompt opposing muscles to contract and release. The muscles attached to tendons tug on bones, causing your body to move as instructed. ▼

Balance problems

Eight million American adults report persistent trouble with balance, according to the National Institutes of Health, and millions more struggle with long-term dizziness. Changes tied to growing older or health issues may underpin these problems. Medications may cause drowsiness, dizziness, or nerve damage. Tight, inflexible, or weak muscles and poor posture impinge on balance, too. And, certainly, a combination of these problems could be at play. Below, you can read about these issues and others in greater detail.

Investigating balance problems

If you frequently feel unsteady on your feet or suffer from dizziness or vertigo (the sensation of spinning), start by talking to your doctor. He or she may propose a physical exam and medication review, plus further testing as needed.

Physical exam

A thorough physical exam can uncover underlying health problems. This is the time to report bothersome symptoms, such as dizziness, vertigo, lightheadedness, blurred vision, or confusion. Sometimes people with balance disorders experience other symptoms, too: nausea and vomiting, heart rate and blood pressure changes, and anxiety or panic. It's important to explain to your doctor when symptoms occur, and whether they are long-lasting or come and go. Any recent illnesses or injuries, particularly from falls, may provide clues, too. For example, even a bad cold can temporarily upset the vestibular system.

Your blood pressure may be taken while you're seated, then measured again immediately after you stand, and possibly a few minutes later. A sudden drop in blood pressure when you change position like this—called orthostatic hypotension—can make you dizzy and increase the risk of falling (see "Blood pressure," page 6).

Report joint stiffness or soreness. Your doctor may check reflexes and range of motion (how far you can move a joint in a given direction), particularly in your lower body. You may be asked to do a few basic balance tests under supervision. A "get up and go test" requires you to rise from a chair without pushing off with your arms, and then walk several steps back and forth. This allows your doctor to assess balance and gait (the speed and rhythm of the way you walk). Taking a few steps with your eyes closed shows whether proprioception is impaired. A basic test of dizziness may be done by moving your head through different positions, which can provide clues about inner ear problems. Tests for peripheral neuropathy, such as the ability to perceive a light touch or vibration on the feet and ankles, may also be done.

Further tests

Depending on what your doctor learns, further evaluation may require a visit to a specialist, such as an otolaryngologist (an ear, nose, and throat specialist, or ENT) or an otologist, a medical doctor who has additional training in hearing and balance disorders. Further testing varies, but may include any of the following:

- **A hearing exam,** which could help point to the underlying problem, since hearing and balance are closely connected in the inner ear. Several relevant tests may be done, according to the Vestibular Disorders Association. For example, an otoacoustic emissions test determines how responsive hair cells lining the cochlea are, and an auditory brainstem response test tracks nerve signals from ear to brain and within different portions of the brain.
- **An electrocardiogram** (ECG) to evaluate the electrical activity of your heart. Irregularities may indicate an arrhythmia, which can cause dizziness and falls, or a problem called syncope, in which blood flow to the brain temporarily slows, which can induce fainting.

- **An echocardiogram** to determine if heart valves are functioning properly.
- **Imaging studies** of the head and brain to look for growths or other abnormalities.
- **A caloric test,** during which warm or cold water is squirted into the ear canal to stimulate the acoustic nerve and balance sensors in the inner ear. Normally this triggers rapid, side-to-side eye movements called nystagmus. The direction of these movements should vary: the eyes should look first toward and then away from the warm water, and away from and then toward the cold water. The response to testing in both ears should be similar. Often, this test is done during videonystagmography or electronystagmography.
- **Videonystagmography,** which uses goggles fitted with infrared cameras to measure eye movements as head position changes. (An older test called electronystagmography captures these movements by using electrodes to measure muscles around the eyes.) A rotational chair may be used with either technique.
- **A computerized dynamic posturography test**, in which you stand on a movable platform. Sensory and motor responses are measured as the platform moves, or as visual patterns change.

Age-related balance problems

A number of changes ascribed to aging get a surprisingly early start: muscle strength begins dwindling in the 30s, for example, and vision declines in the 40s. While you can't sidestep every age-related problem outlined here, you may be able to slow the rate at which some occur, or learn to compensate for changes you can't control. Simply becoming more aware of certain problems may help you stay on your feet, too.

Blood pressure. Most of us worry about high blood pressure, which increases risks for heart attacks and strokes. However, blood pressure may dip suddenly when you stand up, causing dizziness, lightheadedness, blurry vision, and sometimes fainting. Called orthostatic hypotension or postural hypotension, this problem affects as many as one in three elderly people. Possible causes include dehydration, prolonged bed rest, atherosclerosis (the buildup of fatty deposits in arteries), diabetes, and some medications, particularly diuretics and vasodilators used to treat high blood pressure. Treatment varies, depending on the cause. Standing up slowly—sitting first on the side of the bed when you rise, for example—may help.

Hearing and vestibular system. Hearing loss often springs from permanent damage to tiny hair cells in the cochlea. Age and cumulative exposure to loud noise gradually harm these cells. Some die, leaving fewer cells to respond to sounds, thus weakening signals sent to the brain via the auditory nerve. Similarly, hair cells in the vestibular system deteriorate and die off over time, which may affect accurate detection of head position and movement.

Sight. Visual acuity, the ability to focus and see things clearly, diminishes with age. So do depth perception, night vision, and sensitivity to contrast. Various eye problems, from nearsightedness to cataracts, can impair, blur, or distort vision. The loss of visual cues about where you are in terms of your surroundings, which direction you're traveling, and how quickly you're moving compromises balance, forcing you to rely more on other senses. Depending on the problem, corrective lenses or surgery may be necessary. Brighter, nonglare lighting may help, too.

Muscle strength and power. The average 30-year-old can expect to lose 25% of muscle mass and strength by age 70, plus another 25% by age 90. Weaker muscles aren't the whole story, though. A loss of power—which is a function of strength and speed—affects balance, too. Faced with a four-lane intersection, you may have the muscle strength to cross the street. But do you have the muscle power needed to do so before the light turns red? And if you start to trip or lose your balance, power helps you react swiftly. At any age, appropriate exercise can help you rebuild strength and power, or at least slow the pace of decline. Walking and balance workouts that provide plenty of strengthening exercise and explosive bursts of movement (see "Jump! Four moves to help you boost your power," page 16) can help you turn up the power.

Reflexes. The swift, involuntary protective responses known as reflexes tend to slow with age. Thus, it may take more time to react when you start to stumble or if a pet or child scampers underfoot. People also tend to lose some coordination as they grow older. Damage to nerve pathways or disuse due to a sedentary lifestyle can contribute to the problem. Such changes are another important reason to work on developing muscle strength and power.

Proprioception. Knowing where your body is in relation to its surroundings keeps you from stumbling or bumping up against objects. Proprioception may diminish with age, possibly because of peripheral neuropathy, nerve damage that is a long-term complication of diabetes and other conditions, or damage to cells in the inner ear. A cane might help you sense the ground better.

Bones. While bone strength rarely affects balance, it can surely affect the aftermath of a fall. As we grow older, bones become thinner and more fragile. This can lead to osteopenia (low bone mass), which may progress to osteoporosis, a condition that makes bones much more susceptible to breaks. Low calcium and vitamin D intake, hormonal shifts at menopause, a sedentary lifestyle, smoking, too much alcohol, and long-term use of certain medications can accelerate bone loss.

Health conditions that affect balance

A lengthy list of health problems can interfere with balance. This section briefly outlines some of the more common conditions.

Many balance problems, such as those caused by arthritis or milder forms of the eye disorders described below, will respond well to the exercises in the workouts. Milder balance impairments due to stroke, Parkinson's disease, and multiple sclerosis should respond well, too, although these conditions can cause more severe balance problems that are beyond the scope of this report (see "Starting balance workouts safely," page 18). If you're not sure which balance workouts will be helpful for you, talk to your doctor before starting any exercises.

No matter which underlying problems affect your balance, remember that you can do much to prevent dangerous falls by identifying hazards and fixing them, as explained in the checklists starting on page 12.

Vestibular disorders

Ear infections, allergies, head injuries, or problems with blood circulation may temporarily or permanently affect the vestibular system. That sparks trouble with balance, dizziness, and vertigo (the sickening sensation that you or your surroundings are spinning). Treatment varies depending on the disorder. If dizziness and nausea are persistent, vestibular rehabilitation (balance retraining therapy) may be recommended. A trained vestibular rehabilitation therapist can recommend a treatment plan combining certain head, body, and eye exercises, which may help ease these symptoms. Talk to your doctor about this.

Three common vestibular disorders pose particular problems with balance, as follows.

Benign paroxysmal positional vertigo (BPPV). Sometimes the tiny stones called canaliths tumble out of the utricle and into a semicircular canal (see "Vestibular system," page 3). This prevents the cupula and the sensory hair cells inside it from tilting properly, so that conflicting messages about the position of your head are sent to the brain. Turning your head to catch a glimpse behind you or rolling over in bed can cause the dizzy, room-spinning sensation of vertigo. Possible causes of BPPV include head injury and aging. The Epley maneuver, a series of simple movements done while sitting upright, lying down, and turning your head to one side may help shift errant canaliths out of the semicircular canal. This canalith repositioning procedure must be guided by a trained clinician.

Labyrinthitis. When the labyrinth is infected or swollen, temporary dizziness and loss of balance may occur. An upper respiratory tract ailment like tonsillitis, sinusitis, a cold, or an ear infection is often the culprit. Allergies, smoking, alcohol use, stress, and fatigue can increase the risk of developing labyrinthitis. Washing your hands often and getting an annual flu shot can help stave off certain infections that contribute to it.

Ménière's disease. Hearing and balance are affected by this condition, which occurs mainly in women over 40. Endolymph builds up in the inner ear to the point where it ruptures the membranes that hold it, damaging the surrounding sensory cells. Spells of Ménière's disease come and go, lasting minutes or hours, and triggering hearing loss, vertigo, and tinnitus (persistent ringing or other noise in the ears). Sometimes this disorder stops on its own; in other cases, sufferers need medication or surgery for relief. Cutting down on salt (sodium) in your diet and limiting alcohol or caffeine can lessen the dizziness. Sometimes diuretics are used, too.

Eye disorders

Eye disorders can blur or distort sight or even punch holes in your field of vision. When sight is impaired, balance suffers. Two eye disorders—glaucoma and diabetic retinopathy—are especially common culprits. Initially, glaucoma diminishes peripheral vision. If left untreated, it leads to increasing blindness. Diabetic retinopathy can lead to blurred central vision and spots and floaters that create holes in the field of vision.

Arthritis

Stiff, sore joints hamper movement. If your ankles or knees are arthritic, for example, it's hard to bend them, which affects your ability to balance and react when you trip. If your neck is stiff, your range of motion—how far you can move in any direction—is limited, so that you tend to move your upper body to look behind you. This can upset your balance, too. One study of seniors found that those reporting lower limb arthritis, as compared to those who did not, were 22% more likely to have fallen during a 12-month period. What's more, researchers noted, they performed worse on tests of knee and ankle muscle strength, lower limb proprioception, and certain measures of balance.

Peripheral neuropathy

This disorder may impede balance by impairing proprioception and muscle strength, as well as through the distracting quality of pain. Throughout the peripheral nervous system, signals shuttle toward the central nervous system, which sends instructions back to varied players in the neural network. Motor nerves control conscious movements, sensory nerves report sensations like touch and pain, and autonomic nerves regulate essential, unconscious biological functions, such as breathing and digestion. Damaged motor or sensory nerves, for example, cause a variety of unpleasant symptoms, such as muscle weakness; shooting pains; burning; or numbness, tingling, and prickling sensations called paresthesias.

Often, nerve fibers farthest from the central nervous system—in the feet and legs, or hands and arms—malfunction first. Over 100 kinds of neuropathy have been identified. These ailments may be short-lived, lasting only until damaged nerves heal, or progress slowly and permanently.

Heart arrhythmia

A hindrance in the speed or rhythm of the heartbeat called an arrhythmia may interfere with blood supply to the brain, spurring sudden weakness, lightheadedness, or dizziness that affects balance, or more serious problems like fainting or a heart attack.

Stroke

Strokes occur when a blocked blood vessel suddenly interrupts the flow of oxygen and nutrients to part of the brain, or, less often, when a blood vessel bursts inside the brain. The compromised brain cells die off, causing many serious problems that can affect balance, including weakness, numbness, trouble seeing, trouble walking, dizziness, and loss of coordination. Often, the physical deficits are confined to one side of the body, but stroke can wreak havoc with thought processes and attention that play into balance, too.

Parkinson's disease

Cells in certain areas of the brain produce dopamine. This naturally occurring neurotransmitter regulates movement, among other tasks. The loss of these brain cells causes Parkinson's disease, which affects the system of motor nerves throughout the body. This condition impairs balance in a variety of ways: through tremors in the legs and other parts of the body, rigidity of the limbs and trunk, slowness of movement called bradykinesia, and direct hindrance of systems affecting balance and coordination. Difficulty walking occurs as the disease progresses.

Multiple sclerosis (MS)

This unpredictable central nervous system condition disrupts communication between brain and body.

Good posture counts

By standing up straight, you center your weight over your feet. This helps you balance properly. Good posture also helps you maintain correct form while exercising, which results in fewer injuries and greater gains.

Poor posture doesn't just stem from a habit of slumping. Inflexibility feeds into it as well. As muscles tighten up, they shorten. This curtails range of motion—that is, how far a joint can move in a given direction. The muscles known as hip flexors, for example, allow you to bend at the hip and bring your knee up toward your chest. Overly tight, short-ened hip flexors tug your upper body forward and disrupt your posture. Likewise, overly tight chest muscles can pull your shoulders forward. Unless you do stretches to counter muscle tightening, your range of motion is likely to become increasingly limited as time passes.

Muscle strength matters for posture, too. The so-called core muscles of the back, side, pelvis, and buttocks form a sturdy central link between your upper and lower body. Weak core muscles encourage slumping, which tips your body forward and thus off-balance. Strong lower leg muscles help keep you from swaying too much while standing.

Our balance workouts address these problems with exercises that build strength where it counts and stretches that loosen up tight muscles. We recommend quick posture checks in the mirror before and during balance exercises. Cultivating aware-ness and buffing core strength and flexibility can help you improve your posture noticeably over the course of weeks.

Good posture means
- chin parallel to the floor
- shoulders even (roll your shoulders up, back, and down to help achieve this)
- neutral spine (no flexing or arching to overemphasize the curve in your lower back)
- arms at your sides with elbows straight and even
- abdominal muscles braced
- hips even
- knees even and pointing straight ahead
- feet pointing straight ahead
- body weight distributed evenly on both feet.

If you're seated, not standing, keep your chin parallel to the floor, your shoulders, hips, and knees at even heights, and your knees and feet pointing straight ahead.

It often causes muscle weakness and interferes with balance and coordination, sometimes making walk-ing, or even standing, difficult or impossible. As MS advances, it can cause partial or complete paralysis. A variety of other possible symptoms may interfere with balance, too: dizziness; tremors; trouble with concen-tration and attention; and pain, numbness, prickling, or "pins and needles" sensations.

Medications that affect balance

By keeping blood sugar at safe levels, hearts thump-ing rhythmically, and moods afloat, medications can be lifesaving. Yet side effects and interactions from prescription and nonprescription drugs may increase your fall risk in numerous ways, according to the Centers for Disease Control and Prevention. Prime examples include blurred vision, dizziness or lightheadedness stemming from low blood pres-sure, drowsiness, delirium, and impaired alertness or judgment. Some medications may damage the inner ear, spurring temporary or permanent bal-ance disorders.

Which drugs raise the risk for falling?

Often, it's the sheer number of medicines taken, rather than a single drug, that causes problems. According to a national health survey, a third of 45- to 64-year-olds, and two-thirds of people 65 and older, take three or more prescription drugs over the course of a month. Earlier findings suggested 40% of older adults living on their own took five or more drugs per day, and 12% took more than 10 drugs per day. Some gerontologists say they rarely see patients who take fewer than six or seven. Taking many medications at the same time can boost the severity and frequency of side effects among people of any age. Older adults are especially vulner-able, because people's bodies absorb and respond to drugs differently with age.

While it's true that some medicines are more likely to play a role in falls than others, many of these drugs are surprisingly difficult to avoid. A Swedish study published in the *Journal of the American Geriatrics Society* looked at changes in medications six months before and six months after a hip fracture among people ages 60 or older. Before the hip fracture occurred, two-thirds of study participants had been taking at least one drug known to increase fall risk, such as those described below. Yet the proportion of participants taking these drugs after the fracture rose to nearly 98%, largely because of substantial rises in treatment for heart problems, pain, and depression.

The lengthy list of drugs that increase fall risk includes but is not limited to the following:

- antidepressant drugs, such as tricyclic antidepressants, selective serotonin reuptake inhibitors (SSRIs), serotonin-norepinephrine reuptake inhibitors (SNRIs), and monoamine oxidase inhibitors (MAOIs)
- anti-anxiety drugs, such as benzodiazepines
- anticholinergic/antispasmodic drugs
- antihistamines
- blood pressure drugs, such as diuretics, alpha blockers, centrally acting antihypertensives, ACE inhibitors, angiotensin-receptor blockers (ARBs), and beta blockers (including eye drops)
- heart drugs, such as antiarrhythmics, nitrates and other vasodilators, and digoxin
- pain drugs, such as opioids and nonsteroidal anti-inflammatory drugs (NSAIDs)
- sleep drugs, such as sedatives and hypnotics.

Generally, it's wise to keep the number of medications you take to a minimum. Routinely discussing your medications with your doctor is the best way to ensure this.

How your doctor can help

If you are experiencing side effects that could make falls more likely, ask your primary care doctor or gerontologist to do a medication review. Put all your prescription and nonprescription medications and supplements in a bag, and bring them with you to this visit—or at least bring a complete and up-to-date list, including dosages and how often you take each one. It's best to carry such a list with you at all times, anyway, in case of an emergency. For the purposes of the review, however, it's likely to be more accurate if you bring everything with you, as people tend to leave things off the list, especially supplements and the doses they take.

Your doctor may consider different strategies, such as the following.

Prune the list. Medications tend to multiply, especially if you see several doctors. One specialist may put you on a drug, unaware that another physician has prescribed a similar drug—or perhaps one that causes an adverse interaction. Your doctor can review the list to make sure you still need these drugs and get rid of any you don't need.

Consider a lower dose. This can be especially helpful in reducing side effects from diuretics and cardiovascular drugs. Of course, don't alter dosages yourself. Your doctor should determine whether it is safe and effective to change a dose.

Substitute a drug. Sometimes it's possible to switch to a drug with different side effects.

Change the time of day a drug is taken. For example, taking all your blood pressure medications first thing in the morning may cause your blood pressure to drop too low, increasing your risk of falls. Your doctor might suggest that you separate your blood pressure pills, taking some in the morning and some in the evening.

Take a different tack. Sometimes, lifestyle changes work well enough to enable you to lower the dose of a medication or eliminate it entirely. You might be able to apply relaxation techniques and sleep hygiene tips that allow you to safely taper off sleep medication, for instance. Or stepping up exercise and eating better may permit you to take lower doses of diabetes and blood pressure drugs. Weight loss can often reduce or eliminate the need for blood pressure and diabetes pills, and it also eases the strain on knees and hips. ◗

Preventing falls

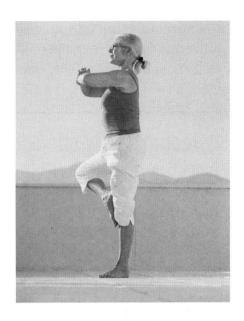

Occasional scrapes, bangs, and bruises from falls are a fact of life from the day we're born. Consequences grow worse as we age, however. Falls tend to occur more often, too. Among people 65 and older, falling ranks as the top cause of injuries. Millions of these nonfatal injuries are serious enough to merit a trip to the emergency room. Worse, fall injuries prove fatal in 10 out of 100,000 cases among 65- to 74-year-olds, and in 147 out of 100,000 falls in those ages 85 and older.

Why do people fall?

Often, falls occur when a combination of risk factors collide. Some risks are extrinsic, meaning that they have to do with the environment around you: for example, broken pavement, a slick area of ice or wet floor, clutter, dim lighting that hides obstacles, the rolled edge of a rug. Others are intrinsic—that is, specific to you: your vision and corrective eyewear; your muscle strength, power, and flexibility; any health problems or medicines that affect balance; and even the shoes or slippery socks on your feet.

To prevent falls, then, it makes sense to address both types of problems. In 2010, a major U.S. Preventive Services Task Force review of the evidence noted that the most promising strate-gies for addressing intrinsic issues were exercise or physical therapy, which reduced fall risk by 13%, and, more surprisingly, vitamin D supplements (with or without cal-

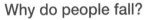

Fear of falling

Worrying persistently about taking a fall leads some people to act more cautious as they make their daily rounds. Others pull back entirely from a range of activities still well within their abilities. Such a pronounced fear of falling can exist even if no such spill has occurred.

Fear of falling chips away zest in life, self-confidence, and well-being. Social isolation, anxiety, and depression may follow. Physical abilities may wane as well. Ironically, having a fear of falling is actually associated with greater risk of suffering future falls.

What helps ease fear of falling? Tai chi, a form of exercise that involves moving gently through a series of poses, has shown promise in a few studies, yet had no real effect in others. Common sense, as well as research evidence, suggests a two-pronged approach—physical and psychological—might make the difference. In one study of 186 adults ages 60 or older, participants scored lowest on fear of falling and highest on mobility and quality of life if they received a combination of two therapies—intensive tai chi plus a program of cognitive behavioral therapy (CBT) aimed at encouraging the view that fall risk and falls were controllable. The training lasted for eight weeks, and participants were tested five months later. Among participants who did neither tai chi nor CBT, fear of falling actually increased. Larger, multisite studies with a longer follow-up period are needed to confirm these findings.

cium), which cut fall risk by 17%. One important study in the journal *BMJ* found that 700 to 1,000 international units (IU) of vitamin D taken daily cut falling risk by 19%, and some evidence suggests that 700 to 800 IU of vitamin D a day also reduces hip fractures. Smaller doses did not have this same effect. Check with your doctor about the most effective dose of vitamin D for you.

There are no clinical trials testing extrinsic strategies, but certainly, clearing clutter, installing grab rails in the shower, tying shoelaces properly, and similar safety steps remain wise.

Personal safety checklist

 As an old adage tells us, an ounce of prevention is worth a pound of cure. Start by performing this safety inventory of your physical condition and habits to identify potential hazards. Circle any items that raise your personal risk for falls. Then take action to solve problems one by one. Balance training, which is covered in depth in the workouts in this report, is a big part of the solution, too.

Posture
Poor posture can throw your body off balance.

☐ **Actions:** Practice posture checks (see "Good posture counts," page 9). The stretches and core strength exercises in the balance workouts can help, too.

Eyes
Eyesight less than 20/60, cataracts, decreasing depth perception, and reduced sensitivity to contrast—all of which can be detected in a standard eye exam—contribute to falls. So do eye disorders like glaucoma, macular degeneration, and diabetic retinopathy, which affect your field of vision.

☐ **Actions:** Have your eyes tested annually. Discuss options for correcting your vision with an eye specialist. Wear appropriate corrective eyewear.

Eyewear
Reading glasses, bifocals, trifocals, and progressive lenses are enormously helpful in correcting vision, but they can be hazardous when you're walking. If you look straight ahead as you walk, these lenses blur objects scattered on the floor or ground, making it hard to see possible hazards. One study found people who wore reading glasses regularly were twice as likely to fall as those who did not wear them.

☐ **Actions:** Save reading glasses for close work only. Consider buying a pair of glasses with single-vision distance lenses for activities like walking outdoors.

If you do choose to wear bifocals, trifocals, or progressive lenses, be aware of the dangers. Talk to an eye specialist about your options.

Muscles
Loss of muscle strength and power—particularly in the lower body—erodes balance, setting the stage for falls and making it hard to catch yourself if you do trip. Tight, shortened muscles limit your range of motion, too.

☐ **Actions:** Exercise can improve strength, power (see "Jump! Four moves to help you boost your power," page 16), reflexes, and balance, while stretches enhance flexibility. Get the exercise you need to stay strong and healthy through balance workouts, walking, and other activities described in this report.

Stiff, sore joints
Stiff joints limit movement and make it harder to catch yourself if you do trip. If you have trouble turning your neck, for example,

you tend to turn your upper body to look behind you, which can throw you off balance. Pain itself takes attention away from walking or moving safely.

☐ **Actions:** Discuss ways to ease painful, swollen joints with your doctor. Strengthening exercises and stretches will help, too, according to the Arthritis Foundation.

Ankles

Weak ankles or stiff, inflexible ankle joints make walking harder. Stumbles may occur more when the rear foot doesn't clear the ground properly, making the toes more likely to catch against the ground as you try to move forward.

☐ **Actions:** Stretches and strengthening exercises shown in the balance workouts in this report will help.

Feet

Foot pain or numbness may make falls more likely.

☐ **Actions:** Discuss options for easing pain with your doctor (see "Links between pain and falls," page 14). Call your doctor if you notice pain, burning, or numbness in your feet.

Shoes

High heels, slip-on shoes, loose slippers, and smooth, slippery soles may promote falls.

☐ **Actions:** Wear sturdy shoes, preferably with low or flat heels and nonskid, rubber soles. Oxford-style laced shoes or sneakers are good bets.

Health problems

Blood pressure fluctuations, heart problems, inner ear disorders, and nerve damage are among the ailments that contribute to falls (see "Health conditions that affect balance," page 7).

☐ **Actions:** Consult your doctor if you suffer dizziness or other balance problems.

Medications

Many medications cause dizziness or drowsiness that can precede a fall (see "Medications that affect balance," page 9).

☐ **Actions:** Report dizziness or drowsiness to your doctor. Discuss whether changing medications or lowering dosages might help. Bring medications and supplements (or a list detailing these) to doctor's visits.

Alcohol use

Alcohol impairs judgment, slows reaction time, and cranks up clumsiness—a veritable recipe for falls. As people age, it takes less alcohol to prompt such problems. Mixing medications and alcohol can exacerbate side effects like dizziness or drowsiness. Additionally, alcohol raises the risk for developing the inner ear disorders labyrinthitis and Ménière's disease (see "Vestibular disorders," page 7). Alcoholism is also one cause of peripheral neuropathy (see page 8), which also affects balance.

☐ **Actions:** Avoid or limit alcohol. This is especially important if you take medication or have labyrinthitis or Ménière's disease. Be aware of how alcohol affects you if you do drink.

Weight

Excess weight can cause shortness of breath and gait problems that may affect your center of balance. Being overweight or obese also puts painful strain on your knees and hips. (Just walking across level ground requires the knees to support up to one-and-a-half times your body weight; when going up or down stairs, each knee bears two to three your times body weight.) In addition, it increases your risk for developing osteoarthritis of the knee, which in turn can cause changes in gait as well as sudden pain that can make you lurch or lose your balance.

☐ **Actions:** You can reduce pressure on the knee by strengthening quadriceps muscles on the front of your thighs through regular balance workouts and daily walks, if possible. Better yet, try to reach a healthier weight by combining these workouts with a healthy diet.

Links between pain and falls

Pain is a constant companion for people who live with arthritis, lower back problems, neuropathy, and other uncomfortable chronic conditions. Using data gathered for the MOBILIZE Boston study, which is following roughly 750 adults ages 70 or older living in the surrounding community, researchers considered whether pain plays a role in falls.

For a year and a half, participants completed monthly calendar cards, marking down whether they had fallen and the average amount of pain they had experienced during that month. During the study period, 55% of participants fell at least once. Writing in *The Journal of the American Medical Association*, the researchers reported that falls were more common among those who complained of two or more painful sites on the body or more severe pain at the start of the study.

Whether better pain relief could help reduce falls is a question for a randomized controlled study. Possibly, some pain-easing medications may cause dizziness or drowsiness that could be counterproductive. Equally intriguing is the question of how pain contributes to falls. The researchers speculated on a few possibilities: by weakening muscles, by slowing nerve and muscle response, by creating a distraction, or by derailing mental resources that would normally help a person avoid a fall or recover from a stumble.

Until more information is forthcoming from studies, easing pain seems a worthwhile goal. To that end, you can take these steps:

- Work with your doctor to better control pain. Be aware of any dizziness or drowsiness from medications, though, and report it to your doctor. Choosing the right type and level of pain relief may require some trial and error.

- Seek ways to reduce pain other than medication. Acupuncture shows promise in easing chronic low back pain and osteoarthritis of the knee. Gentle self-massage and applications of cold or heat may help, though this depends on the underlying problem causing your pain. Explore these and other options with your doctor to be sure they fit your situation.

- Exercise can help reduce some forms of chronic pain. However, you may need to avoid repetitive or jarring movements, such as running or even too much walking. Water aerobics, the flowing movements of tai chi, gentle yoga moves (see "Yoga Balance Workout," page 43), and low-impact exercises, such as those in the Beginner Balance Workout, may be better choices. If your pain results from arthritis, try the two-hour pain rule recommended by the Arthritis Foundation. Some short-lived discomfort is likely when you exercise, especially if you haven't been active. However, if you feel more pain two hours after you finish exercising than before you started, you probably overdid it. Pare back to the point where this is no longer true (for example, by walking less or doing fewer reps or sets of balance exercises). Then, step up your level of exercise very gradually, keeping the rule in mind.

- Be sure your footwear is as comfortable and supportive as possible. Adding cushions for tender spots and orthotics to properly position your foot may help. See a podiatrist, if necessary.

If you do suffer from chronic pain, be aware that it is a powerful distraction. It could make you more likely to slip or trip in unknown, uneven, or dimly lit surroundings. So, good lighting, clearing away obstacles, and trying to focus attention when walking are especially important for you.

Home safety checklist

Do an annual room-by-room safety inventory of your home. That will help you spot hazards that should be addressed. By reviewing this list periodically, you can make updates as your needs change.

Bedrooms

☐ Keep a phone and lamp close to your bed. Lamps that turn on at a touch are easy to manage.

☐ A firm mattress helps with balance as you rise from the bed. Make sure the bed is low enough that you can put your feet flat on the floor when you're sitting on the edge.

☐ Arrange furniture so that the path to the door is clear.

☐ If you use a cane or walker, keep it within easy reach when you go to bed.

Bathrooms

☐ Install night lights.

☐ Install grab bars and nonslip mats or adhesive safety strips in the bathtub or shower.

☐ If you have trouble sitting down on the toilet, install an elevated seat with armrests.

☐ If the floor is slippery when wet, consider installing textured tiles to help prevent falls.

☐ If tub height is a problem, consider installing a low-threshold shower.

Kitchen

☐ Store often-used items where you can easily reach them.

☐ Keep a sturdy step stool handy to reach items in high cabinets.

Entrances and hallways

☐ All outside doors should have lights.

☐ Outside walkways should be free of cracks, holes, and clutter. Repair any rotted or crumbling steps.

☐ Mats inside the door should lie flat and have a nonskid backing.

☐ Hallways should be well lit.

Stairways

☐ Make sure there is a light switch at the top and bottom of the stairway.

☐ Install a handrail that runs the full length of the stairs.

☐ Keep stairs in good repair and clear of clutter.

☐ Stair carpeting, if any, should be tacked down tightly.

Housewide

☐ Keep floors clutter-free.

☐ Keep electric cords tucked out of the way.

☐ Make sure you can turn on lights without walking into rooms.

☐ Lighting should be even, with no splashes of shadow or glare. Add task lights where needed.

☐ Skip scatter rugs, if possible. All carpeting should lie flat and have nonskid backing.

☐ Program emergency numbers into phones.

☐ If door thresholds create tripping hazards, replace them with lower thresholds (a quarter-inch if edges are square; or a half-inch if edges are slanted). ◗

Activities that enhance balance

Activities that challenge balance while holding steady (static balance) or moving (dynamic balance) are familiar forms of balance training. Standing with one foot in front of another, lifting a foot off the floor, and shifting weight in various directions are three examples offered by the American College of Sports Medicine (ACSM).

Experts at ACSM note that balance training can be made progressively harder by reducing your base of support—instead of standing on two legs, stand on one leg—and later adding dynamic moves that shift your center of gravity, such as walking forward by putting one foot directly in front of the other, as you would on a balance beam. When you're ready to raise the bar further, you can move from a flat, stable surface like the floor to a soft, rounded, or otherwise less stable surface. The instability forces you to work harder at maintaining balance. Another advanced challenge is reducing sensory input by closing your eyes (keeping a sturdy chair nearby to steady yourself).

Most likely, you already engage in some activities that help hone balance, especially if you're an active person. Many of the balance-enhancing activities noted below are included in our workouts.

- **Walking, biking, and climbing stairs** strengthen muscles in your lower body. (Using a recumbent bike or stair stepper is an option when balance is compromised.)
- **Resistance exercises** build muscle strength. Resistance can be supplied by body weight, free

Jump! Four moves to help you boost your power

When you start to stumble, quick muscle reactions can save you from a fall. Yet with age and disuse, the nerve-signaling system for muscles starts to deteriorate. Fast-twitch muscle fibers, which supply bursts of power for quick motion, are lost at a greater rate than slow-twitch fibers, which are called upon most for endurance activities like walking. Preliminary studies on power training suggest movements designed to restore nerve pathways can help with this.

The power training moves suggested below are safe for most people who are reasonably steady on their feet. There are exceptions, however. If you have osteoporosis, check with your doctor to be sure that these jumps won't hurt your bones. If your balance is poor, it's best to focus on improving it first with the balance workouts that are safest for you, such as the Beginner Balance Workout.

1 **Easy jump:** Jumps are excellent power moves because they call for quick, explosive energy. Start with an easy jump. Stand in front of a kitchen counter, feet together and four fingers on each hand (no thumbs) lightly touching the counter for support. Slightly bend your knees to gather energy, then jump in place, rising just a few inches off the floor. Try to land softly with bent knees. Do 5–10 reps.

2 **Lateral jump:** A more advanced version without support is a lateral jump. Put a strip of masking tape on the floor. Stand up straight to the right of the tape, with your feet hip-width apart and arms at your sides. Slightly bend your knees to gather energy. Then jump to the left, up and over the tape. Steady yourself. Slightly bend your knees, and jump back over the tape to the right. This completes one rep. Do 5–10 reps.

Two more power moves, described below, are based on exercises in the "Beginner Balance Workout" beginning on page 25. The difference is that you change tempo so that you move fast in the first half of the movement and slower in the second half. To be sure you do these exercises correctly, check the tips and techniques described in the workout.

3 **Heel raises:** While holding on to the back of a sturdy chair, quickly lift up onto the balls of your feet in one count. Hold for two counts. Slowly lower your heels back to the floor for three counts. Do 10 reps.

4 **Stand up, sit down:** Sit in a sturdy chair with your hands crossed on your chest or held out in front of you at chest level. Stand up to two counts. Hold for two counts. Slowly sit down with control to four counts. Do 10 reps.

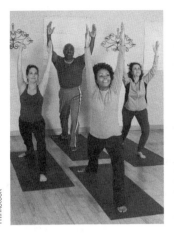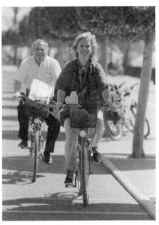

Most types of physical activity can enhance balance in one way or another, according to the American College of Sports Medicine. Yoga and biking are two forms of exercise that help.

weights, elastic bands, or weight machines. Many of the strengthening exercises selected for our workouts focus on hip and leg muscles. Some core muscles are targeted, too, to help improve posture and balance.

- **Stretches** loosen tight muscles, which affect posture and balance.
- **Power training** (see "Jump! Four moves to help you boost your power," page 16) can help keep a momentary stagger from turning into a bad spill.

- **Yoga** strengthens and stretches tight muscles, while challenging static and dynamic balance. There are many styles of yoga. Our Yoga Balance Workout (see page 43) offers a variety of classic poses.
- **Tai chi**—a practice of slow, graceful movements that flow smoothly from one pose to the next and mesh with meditative breathing—is very good for balance. During the choreographed moves, gradual shifts of weight from one foot to another combine with rotating the trunk and extending the limbs in a series of challenges to balance. Like yoga, tai chi strengthens and stretches tight muscles, too.
- **Pilates** challenges static and dynamic balance. It strengthens the full range of core muscles especially well.
- **Sports like tennis, squash, soccer, and golf** build balance. They strengthen lower body muscles, too (assuming you're walking from hole to hole in golf, rather than hopping into a golf cart).

What if you're not at all active? Take heart. Research shows that sedentary people can improve strength and balance dramatically through exercise at any age. Our balance workouts will show you how to make gains safely. ◗

Starting balance workouts safely

Our program aims to help you become steadier on your feet. But before starting the workouts, consider whether you need to call your doctor for a go-ahead or see another expert who can help you work on your balance safely.

Do you need to see a doctor?

As every doctor will tell you, exercise is essential for a healthy life. Generally, light to moderate exercise is safe for healthy adults. Most people—healthy or not—can safely take up walking. But before starting our walking program or the balance workouts, it's best to check in with your doctor if

- you are extremely unsteady on your feet
- you have dizzy spells or take medicine that makes you feel dizzy or drowsy
- you have a chronic or unstable health condition, such as heart disease (or several risk factors for heart disease), asthma or another respiratory ailment, high blood pressure, osteoporosis, or diabetes.

If you are uncertain, you may want to use a helpful tool developed by the Canadian Society for Exercise Physiology. Called the Physical Activity Readiness Questionnaire (PAR-Q), it can help you decide whether to talk to a doctor before embarking on or ramping up any exercise program. You can find it at www.health.harvard.edu/PAR-Q.

If you do need to speak to your doctor, find out if you can follow the specific balance workouts you'd like to try from this report. The Beginner Balance Workout (see page 25) is an easy entry point for practically anyone.

Odds are good that your doctor will feel the easier workouts and walking plan are fine as long as you start gradually, build up slowly, and attend to safety tips—including using a cane or walker, if you normally use one. Or, possibly, your doctor might want to modify certain exercises. If necessary, your doctor can refer you to a physiatrist, physical therapist, or another specialist like a neurologist or cardiologist for further evaluation. Sometimes, it's safest to work out with the supervision of an experienced personal trainer or a health professional, or to choose a supervised class at a hospital or other facility.

Physiatrists, also known as rehabilitation physicians, are board-certified medical doctors who specialize in treating nerve, muscle, and bone conditions that affect movement. Stroke, back problems, Parkinson's disease, neuropathy, and debilitating arthritis or obesity are a few examples. A physiatrist can tailor exercises to enhance recovery after surgery or an injury, or work with limitations posed by pain or problems affecting movement. He or she can also tell you whether certain types of exercise will be helpful or harmful given your specific health history.

Physical therapists help restore abilities to people with health problems or injuries affecting muscles, bones, or nerves. Their expertise can be valuable if you have suffered a lingering sprain or are recovering from a stroke or heart attack. Some specialize in geriatrics, orthopedics, cardiopulmonary rehabilitation, or other areas. After having received a bachelor's degree, physical therapists must graduate from an accredited physical therapy program. Most of these programs offer doctoral degrees. Additionally, they must pass a national exam given by the Federation of State Boards of Physical Therapy and be licensed by their state. Those who specialize complete advanced training and additional national exams to become board certified.

Physical therapy assistants provide physical therapy services under the supervision of a physical therapist. They must complete a two-year associate's degree, pass a national exam, and, in most states, be licensed.

Personal trainers are fitness specialists who can help ensure that you're doing exercises properly.

While encouraging and motivating you, they can teach new skills, fine-tune your form, change up routines to beat boredom, and safely push you to the next level. No nationwide licensing requirements exist for personal trainers, although standards for the accrediting fitness organizations that train them have been set by the National Commission for Certifying Agencies. Two well-respected organizations that offer programs of study for personal trainers are the American College of Sports Medicine (ACSM) and the American Council on Exercise (ACE). Others include the National Council on Strength and Fitness (NCSF), the National Strength and Conditioning Association (NSCA), and the National Academy of Sports Medicine (NASM). All fitness organizations have different requirements for training and expertise. Some trainers specialize in working with particular populations—for example, older adults or athletes—and may have taken courses and possibly certifying exams in these areas.

Additional safety tips

The following tips can also help you use the workouts in this report safely.

Pay attention. If your attention is focused, you'll be less likely to fall. Before you start your exercises, use the bathroom, so an uncomfortably full bladder or imminent accident won't distract you. (If necessary, wear a pad when exercising to ease worry about accidents.)

Stay safe. If you need a cane or walker to steady yourself, use it. If not, you can steady yourself with a sturdy chair or counter, or by standing in a corner of the room. If you feel dizzy while exercising, sit down until the feeling passes.

Do the warm-ups. Prepare your body for the workout by following the instructions in "Warm-ups" on page 24.

Wear the right outfit. Choose comfortably padded sneakers or walking shoes with rubber soles. If you'll be walking outside, wear layers for cool weather, plus a hat, sunscreen, and sunglasses, as needed.

Go slow. Hurrying or pushing yourself too hard can cause accidents. Initially, less is better: consider doing fewer repetitions or an easier variation of an exercise the first time you try it.

Brace yourself. Practice bracing yourself by contracting your abdominal muscles as you stand or sit up straight. Imagine that you are preparing to counter a push on the shoulder from the front, side, or back. When you do balance exercises, you'll use this skill to help keep your balance.

Drink water. Dehydration contributes to dizziness, weakness, heart rhythm disturbances, and low blood pressure. Throughout the day and before exercising, make sure you drink enough water to stay hydrated. Sip water during workouts and walks, too. If you find this means you need a bathroom break, take it before you have to hurry. A fall may be more likely when you're in a rush. ◗

Balance workouts and your overall fitness plan

Better balance is important for avoiding injuries. But to maintain your overall health, you need to engage in physical activity on a regular basis. This chapter offers insight into current exercise guidelines and explains how the balance training program in this Special Health Report dovetails with those.

Current exercise recommendations

You can reap a remarkable list of health benefits by following the current U.S. physical activity guidelines.

- All adults—including people with various disabilities—should aim to spread throughout each week a total of 150 minutes of moderate aerobic activity, or 75 minutes of vigorous activity, or an equivalent mix of the two. (Twenty minutes of moderate activity is roughly equal to 10 minutes of vigorous activity.) During moderate activities, you can talk, but not sing; during vigorous activities, you can manage only a few words aloud without pausing to breathe. You can gain additional health benefits by increasing to 300 minutes of moderate activity,

▶ A walking plan: Simple steps to better balance

Building lower-body strength helps improve balance. Walks can help you do so safely, and they count toward your aerobic activity goals. If health problems make walks especially difficult for you, discuss your options with a physiatrist or physical therapist. Swimming or using specific exercise machines may be a better choice.

Our walking plan (at right) is designed to safely boost physical activity whether you're sedentary or fairly active. The minutes count, not the miles. Here's how to tailor the plan to your needs.

If you aren't in the habit of exercising: Start at the beginning, with Week 1. If you normally use a cane or walker, be sure to do so. You may advance more slowly by repeating levels for a week or longer, as needed.

If you're already exercising: Start at the level that best matches your current routine and build from there. If it helps, you can divide daily walking time into 10-minute chunks (three chunks equals 30 minutes). You may add walking time more quickly if the plan seems too easy. Once you're in shape,

Week	Sessions per week	Daily minutes of brisk walking	Total weekly minutes
Week 1	2	5	10
Week 2	3	5	15
Week 3	4	5	20
Week 4	5	5	25
Week 5	5	10	50
Week 6	5	20	100
Week 7	5	25	125
Week 8	5	30	150

feel free to change time and days while still aiming for at least 150 minutes of walking per week.

If you're looking for more of a challenge: Add time, distance, or hills to improve endurance.

Step by step

1. Begin walking at a slow pace for several minutes to warm up.

2. After that, aim for a brisk walking pace if you can safely manage it. A brisk pace makes singing difficult, but you should be able to talk (see Table 1, page 23). Another way to gauge pace is to count steps per minute with a watch and pedometer. Provided you're walking on level ground, you can use this guide to gauge your pace:

- **Slow** = 80 steps per minute
- **Moderate** (brisk) = 100 steps per minute
- **Brisk** = 120 steps per minute
- **Race walking** = More than 120 steps per minute

3. After you walk, your muscles will be nicely warmed up. This is a good time to do a balance workout or stretches.

or 150 minutes of vigorous activity, or a mix.

- Twice-weekly strengthening activities for all major muscle groups (legs, hips, back, abdomen, chest, shoulders, and arms) are recommended, too.
- Balance exercises—such as the ones in this Special Health Report—are recommended for older adults at risk of falling.
- Flexibility exercises may be helpful.

If this much activity isn't possible for you, experts suggest doing as much as you can. Some activity is always better than none. Even short stints of activity, such as five minutes of walking several times a day, are a good first step toward meeting a larger goal.

The health benefits of exercise

Put simply, staying active helps you feel, think, and look better. Regular exercise can take a load off aching joints by strengthening muscles and chiseling away excess pounds while easing swelling and pain. It allows some people to cut back on medications they take, such as drugs for high blood pressure or diabetes. And that can ease unwelcome side effects and save money.

Strong evidence from thousands of studies shows that engaging in regular exercise

- tacks years onto your life
- helps prevent falls that can lead to debilitating fractures and loss of independence
- lowers your risks for early death, heart disease, stroke, type 2 diabetes, high blood pressure, and metabolic syndrome (a complex problem that blends three or more of the following factors: high blood pressure, high triglycerides, low HDL cholesterol, a large waistline, and difficulty regulating blood sugar)
- promotes cardiovascular health by improving your balance of blood lipids (HDL, LDL, and triglycerides), which in turn helps prevent plaque buildup; helping arteries stay resilient despite aging; bumping up the number of blood vessels feeding the heart; reducing inflammation; and discouraging the formation of blood clots that can block coronary arteries
- lessens the likelihood of getting colon cancer and breast cancer
- helps keep you from gaining weight

- may help with weight loss when combined with the proper diet, which may help slow, or even reverse, knee problems
- eases depression
- boosts mental sharpness in older adults.

Emerging evidence suggests that regular exercise also

- improves functional abilities in older adults—that is, being able to walk up stairs or through a store as you do your shopping, heft groceries, rise from a chair without help, and perform a multitude of activities that permit independence or bring joy to your life
- helps lessen abdominal obesity, which plays a role in many serious ailments, including heart disease, diabetes, and stroke
- boosts bone density (provided the exercises are weight-bearing, meaning they work against gravity)
- lowers the risk for hip fractures
- promotes better sleep
- may lower the risk for Alzheimer's disease
- lowers risks for lung cancer and endometrial cancer.

Fitting balance workouts into an overall exercise plan

Both the balance workouts and our walking plan (see "A walking plan," page 20) are part of your balance training. The walking plan can also help you fulfill your aerobic activity requirements. It ramps up slowly and safely. By week 8, you'll meet the guidelines for aerobic exercise explained above.

Aim to do the balance workout you've chosen two to three times a week. Our workouts emphasize exercises that strengthen legs, hips, and certain core muscles. Stretches help with flexibility. And, of course, every workout focuses on enhancing balance.

So, by following our routine you'll be meeting most of the requirements in the U.S. exercise guidelines. Additional exercises to strengthen your chest, back, abdominal muscles, arms, and shoulders will help you meet the twice-weekly strength exercise guidelines. If you're not sure which strength exercises to add, see the Resources section (page 47) for other Harvard Medical School Special Health Reports that discuss strength training. ◗

Using the workouts

In this chapter, you'll find a list of equipment that you'll need for our workouts, explanations of terms used in the workouts, and answers to common questions. A chart (see Table 1, page 23) describes cues to help you measure the intensity of various activities, including walking.

Choosing the right equipment

Our balance workouts can be done either at home or at the gym. Check each workout description to see what equipment you'll need. Several require no more than a sturdy chair. Others require some of the equipment listed below. (When equipment is listed as optional, that means it's for an easier or harder variation of certain exercises.)

Beamfit beam. This is a five-foot-long balance beam made of lightweight, high-density foam that sits directly on the floor. Only two inches high and six inches wide, it stores easily in a closet. The padded, elevated surface of the beam introduces several elements that make balance exercises more challenging. In a pinch, you can put a strip of masking tape on your floor as a substitute for a balance beam. Since the surface of the floor is stable, this makes the workout intended for the balance beam a bit easier.

Chair. Choose a sturdy chair that won't tip over easily. Unless otherwise noted in the workout description, a plain wooden dining chair without arms or heavy padding works well.

Mat. Choose a well-padded nonslip mat for floor exercises. Yoga mats are readily available. A thick carpet or towels will do in a pinch.

Shoes. Choose a comfortably fitted, rubber-soled shoe with little or no heel for balance exercises. One example is sneakers designed for walking. Walking shoes need to be replaced regularly because they lose support and cushioning over time. Some experts suggest buying new ones every 350 to 550 miles.

Step360. This is a flat platform seated on top of two round, air-filled chambers. When the chambers are full, the platform is more stable. Using less air increases instability, making the workout more challenging.

Yoga strap. This is an inelastic cotton or nylon strap of six feet or longer that helps you position your body properly while doing certain stretches. Choose a strap with a D-ring or buckle fastener on one end. This allows you to put a loop around a foot or leg and then grasp the other end of the strap.

Understanding the workout instructions

When you turn to the workout you've chosen—for instance, the Beginner Balance Workout or the Balance on the Beam Workout—you'll see that each exercise has certain information and instructions, described below:

Repetitions (reps). Each rep is a single complete exercise. It's fine if you can't do all the reps at first. Focus on quality rather than quantity. Good form should always come first. Gradually increase reps as you improve.

Sets. One set is a specific number of repetitions. In our workouts, 10 reps usually add up to a single set. Typically, we suggest doing one to three sets.

Intensity. Intensity measures how hard you work during an exercise. Pay attention to objective physiological cues like breathing, talking, and sweating, or measure intensity through perceived exertion (see Table 1, page 23).

Tempo. This is the count for key movements in an exercise. A 2–2–2 tempo requires you to count to two as you perform a move, hold for two beats, then count to two as you return to the starting position. To avoid hurrying, count while watching or listening to seconds tick by on a clock. When you can no longer maintain the recommended tempo, stop that particular exercise even if you haven't finished all of the reps.

Hold. Hold tells you the number of seconds to pause while holding a pose during an exercise. Many stretches, for example, are held for 10 to 30 seconds. While starting out at 10 seconds is fine, gradually extending that until you can comfortably hold the stretch for 30 seconds will give you better results. So, too, will practicing stretches every day rather than just a few times a week.

Rest. Resting after a set gives your muscles a chance to recharge, which helps you maintain good form. Unless otherwise specified, no rest is needed between sets after stretches or alternating exercises that require you to complete all reps on one leg and then repeat this on the other leg.

Starting position. This describes how to position your body before starting the exercise.

Movement. This explains how to perform one complete repetition correctly.

Tips and techniques. We offer two or three pointers to help you maintain good form and make the greatest gains from the exercise.

Too hard? This gives you an option for making the exercise easier.

Too easy? This gives you an option for making the exercise more challenging.

Neutral is a term you'll notice in the exercises. A neutral spine takes into account the slight natural curves of the spine—don't flex your back or arch it to overemphasize the curve of the lower back. A neutral wrist is firm and straight, not bent upward or downward.

When angles appear in exercise instructions, try visualizing a 90-degree angle as an L or two adjacent sides of a square. To visualize a 30-degree angle, mentally slice the 90-degree angle into thirds, or picture the distance between the minute hand and hour hand of a clock at one o'clock.

Answers to four common questions

The answers to these four frequently asked questions can help you get started on your workouts safely and efficiently.

Table 1: How hard am I working?

Intensity	It feels…	You are…
Light	Easy	Breathing easily Warming up, but not yet sweating Able to talk—or even sing an aria if you have the talent
Light to moderate	You're working, but not too hard	Breathing easily Sweating lightly Still finding it easy to talk or sing
Moderate	You're working	Breathing faster Starting to sweat more Able to talk, not able to sing
Moderate to high	You're really working	Huffing and puffing Sweating Able to talk in short sentences, but concentrating more on exercise than conversation
High	You're working very hard, almost out of gas	Breathing hard Sweating hard Finding talking difficult

1. How can I work out as safely as possible?

Before doing any balance exercises, read the section "Starting balance workouts safely" on page 18. When reading the description of an exercise, pay close attention to the tips and techniques so you can do it properly. Start new exercises cautiously, choosing the easier variation if you like at first to build confidence. (Each exercise has an easier option listed under the heading "Too hard?") Be prepared to catch yourself if you start to wobble: put your hand on a counter or the back of a sturdy chair, or position yourself in the corner of a room so that you can't sway too far without support.

2. Which workout should I do?

Some workouts are much more challenging than others. If you're not completely steady on your feet, first master the Beginner Balance Workout. These are simple, gentle balance exercises that can be done by practically anyone. If you normally need a cane or walker to keep your balance, use it during the workout as well.

Among the more challenging workouts are the Balance in Motion Workout, the Balance 360 Workout, and the Balance on the Beam Workout. Before you try these, build your balancing skills and confidence by mastering easier workouts first.

Pair the workout you choose with the weekly walking program (see "A walking plan," page 20), or other physical activities to give your body the cardio tune-up it needs.

3. What if I can't do all the reps or sets suggested?

Quality and safety are much more important than quantity. Only do as many repetitions as you can manage while following instructions, maintaining good form, and sticking to the specified tempo or holding a pose for the length of time suggested. First, work toward finishing a single set of each exercise. Later, you can gradually add sets up to the number specified as you progress.

4. How often should I do a balance workout?

We recommend doing a full balance workout two to three times a week. Stretches in the balance workouts can be done more often—even daily—to enhance flexibility. Doing a few simple balance exercises (single leg stance, heel raises, side leg lifts, walk the narrow path, and stand up, sit down) during the course of your day can help you improve your balance more quickly. Just be sure to attend to safety.

Warm-ups

If you walk before a balance workout, your muscles are already warmed up. Otherwise, warm up for 5 to 10 minutes before doing exercises by choosing a few of the following standing—or, if necessary, seated—options. If that's too much, a warm shower also counts as a way to warm up muscles. Here are a few warm-up options to pick from:

Standing warm-ups

- Walk a narrow path, one foot in front of the other.
- Lift your knees as you walk.
- Walk on heels.
- Walk on toes.
- Stand for toe taps.
- Stand for knee lifts.
- Dance to a few songs on the radio.

Seated warm-ups

- Roll your shoulders up, back, and down.
- Do knee lifts.
- Rotate your ankles in circles.
- Tap your toes.
- Turn your head right, then left.
- Rotate your wrists in circles.
- Rotate your trunk right, then left.
- Reach up with your right arm, then your left arm. ♥

Beginner Balance Workout

This workout is the perfect first step toward improving shaky balance. It can be done by people of many ages and abilities, including those who are elderly, frail, or recovering from illness or surgery. No equipment other than a sturdy chair or counter is necessary, making this workout excellent for home or travel. If you normally need assistance from a cane or walker to balance, you should use it during this workout.

Focus on good form, rather than worrying about how many repetitions (reps) you can complete. If you find an exercise especially difficult, do fewer reps or try the easier variation. As you improve, try a harder variation. (If this workout is too easy for you, begin with the Standing Balance Workout instead.) Before you start, be sure to read "Starting balance workouts safely," page 18.

Equipment: Sturdy chair or counter.

1 | Shoulder blade squeezes

Reps: 10
Sets: 1
Intensity: Light
Tempo: 2–4–2

Starting position: Sit up tall in a chair. Lift your chest, keeping your shoulders down and back. Brace your abdominal muscles and bend your elbows, palms toward each other.

Movement: While exhaling, roll your shoulders farther down and back, away from your ears. Turn your arms out so your palms face forward, squeezing your shoulder blades together. Hold. Slowly return to starting position.

Tips and techniques:
- Think of squeezing a tennis ball between your shoulder blades.
- Keep your spine neutral and brace your abdominal muscles throughout the movement.
- Breathe comfortably.

Too hard? Squeeze your shoulder blades together gently.

Too easy? Hold squeeze for eight counts and do three sets.

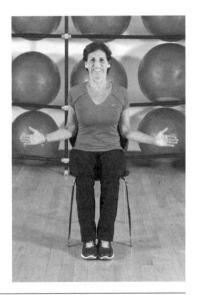

2 | Get up and go

Reps: 10
Sets: 1
Intensity: Moderate
Tempo: Go at your own pace

Starting position: Choosing a path free of obstacles, place a marker (such as a soup can or a small cone) on the floor about 10 feet from a chair. Sit in the chair with your hands on your thighs.

Movement: Stand up and walk forward to the marker. Walk around it and return to the chair. Slowly sit down in the chair.

Tips and techniques:
- After rising from the chair, steady yourself if necessary before walking toward the marker.
- Go at your own pace.
- Breathe comfortably.

Too hard? Use your hands to assist you as you stand up and sit down, or do fewer reps.

Too easy? Pick up your pace.

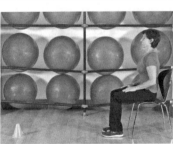

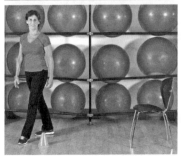

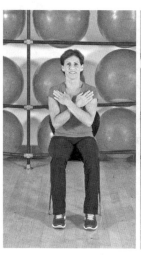
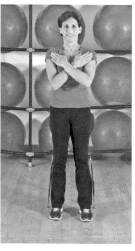

3 | Stand up, sit down

Reps: 10
Sets: 1–3
Intensity: Moderate to high
Tempo: 4–2–4

Starting position: Sit in a chair with your hands crossed on your chest or held out in front of you at chest level.

Movement: Slowly stand up. Hold. Slowly sit down with control.

Tips and techniques:

- Press your heels into the floor and squeeze your buttocks as you stand up to help you balance.

- Steady yourself before you sit down.
- Exhale as you stand, inhale as you sit.

Too hard? Use your hands to assist you as you stand up and sit down, or do fewer reps.

Too easy? Extend your right leg out in front of you with your knee slightly bent, ankle flexed, and heel on the floor. Stand up and sit down. Finish all reps, then repeat with the left leg.

4 | Heel raises

Reps: 10
Sets: 1–3
Intensity: Light to moderate
Tempo: 2–2–2

Starting position: Stand up straight behind a chair, holding the back of it with both hands. Position your feet hip-width apart and evenly distribute your weight on both feet.

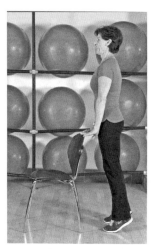

Movement: Lift up on your toes, letting your heels rise off the floor until you're standing on the balls of your feet. Try to balance evenly without allowing your ankles to roll inward or outward. Hold. Lower your heels to the floor, maintaining good posture as you do.

Tips and techniques:

- In the starting position, think of each foot as a room and stand evenly on all four corners. When lifting, try to balance evenly on the front two corners.
- Zip your abdominal muscles up and in as if you were wearing a tight pair of jeans while contracting your buttocks, squeezing your inner thighs, and balancing on the balls of your feet.
- Imagine you have a string at the top of your head pulling you up.

Too hard? Sit down in a chair. Lift your heels off the floor. Hold. Lower your heels to the floor.

Too easy? While holding on to the back of a chair, bend your left knee slightly to lift your foot a few inches off the floor. Do heel lifts with your right foot. Finish all reps, then repeat on the other side.

5 | Standing side leg lift

Reps: 10 on each side
Sets: 1–3
Intensity: Light to moderate
Tempo: 2–2–2

Starting position: Stand up straight behind a chair, holding the back of it with both hands. Put your feet together and evenly distribute your weight on both feet.

Movement: Slowly lift your right leg straight out to the side about 6 inches off the floor. Hold. Return to starting position. Finish all reps, then repeat with the left leg. This completes one set.

Tips and techniques:

- Exhale as you lift your leg.
- Keep your shoulders and hips aligned throughout the exercise.

Too hard? Just touch your foot out to the side on the floor.

Too easy? Hold your leg up for eight counts, or close your eyes.

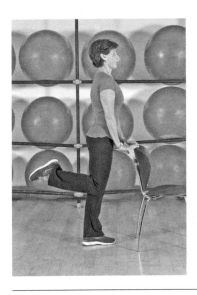

6 | Standing hamstring curls

Reps: 10 on each side
Sets: 1–3
Intensity: Light to moderate
Tempo: 2–2–2

Starting position: Stand up straight behind a chair, holding the back of it with both hands. Extend your right leg behind you with your toes touching the floor.

Movement: Bend your right knee and try to bring the heel toward your right buttock. Hold. Slowly lower your foot to the floor. Finish all reps, then repeat with the left leg. This completes one set.

Tips and techniques:
- Maintain good posture throughout.
- Keep your hips even, squeezing the buttock of the standing leg to help you balance.

Too hard? Lift your leg less, or do fewer reps.

Too easy? Close your eyes.

7 | Seated hamstring stretch

Reps: 3–4
Sets: 1
Intensity: Light to moderate
Hold: 10–30 seconds

Starting position: Sit up tall in a chair.

Movement: Extend your right leg straight in front of you with the heel grounded on the floor and toes pointing to the ceiling. Hinge forward

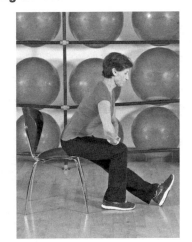

from the hip, placing your hands on your left thigh for support. Keep your spine neutral. Hold. Repeat with the left leg extended. This completes one rep.

Tips and techniques:
- Stretch to the point of mild tension, not pain. You should not feel any pressure behind the knee.
- Relax your shoulders down and back.
- Breathe comfortably.

Too hard? Extend your leg straight in front of you and flex your ankle without hinging forward.

Too easy? Hinge forward from the hip a bit farther into the stretch.

8 | Seated torso rotation

Reps: 3–4
Sets: 1
Intensity: Light
Hold: 10–30 seconds

Starting position: Sit up straight in a chair with your feet flat on the floor, hip-width apart, and arms at your sides.

Movement: Slowly rotate your head and torso to the right side, placing your left hand on the outside of your right knee and your

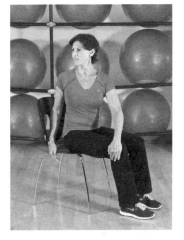

right hand next to your right hip. Hold. Slowly return to starting position. Repeat to the left side, this time with your right hand on the outside of your left knee and your left hand next to your left hip. This completes one rep.

Tips and techniques:
- Sit up straight with chest lifted, abdominal muscles braced, and shoulders down and back.
- Stretch to the point of mild tension, not pain.
- Breathe comfortably.

Too hard? Do not rotate as far.

Too easy? Try to rotate a little bit farther to increase the stretch.

Standing Balance Workout

Another good entry point to balance training, this workout buffs up static balance—that is, the ability to stand in one spot without swaying. If necessary, you can do many of the exercises while holding on to the back of a chair or counter for support, or standing in the corner of a room so that you can touch a wall to steady yourself.

Focus on good form, rather than worrying about how many reps you can complete. If you find an exercise especially difficult, do fewer reps or try the easier variation. As you improve, try a harder variation. Before you start, be sure to read "Starting balance workouts safely," page 18.

Equipment: Sturdy chair (optional), counter (optional), yoga strap (optional).

1 | Heel raises

Reps: 10
Sets: 1–3
Intensity: Light to moderate
Tempo: 2–2–2

Starting position: Stand up straight, feet hip-width apart and weight distributed evenly on both feet. Put your arms at your sides.

Movement: Lift up on your toes until you're standing on the balls of your feet. Try to balance evenly without allowing your ankles to roll inward or outward. Hold. Lower your heels to the floor, maintaining good posture as you do.

Tips and techniques:
- In the starting position, think of each foot as a room and stand evenly on all four corners. When lifting, try to balance evenly on the front two corners.
- Zip your abdominal muscles up and in as if you were wearing a tight pair of jeans and contract your buttocks as you stand on the balls of your feet.
- Imagine you have a string at the top of your head pulling you up.

Too hard? Hold on to a back of a chair or counter.

Too easy? Hold for eight counts.

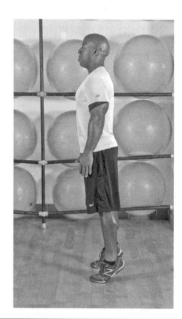

2 | Tandem standing

Reps: 1
Sets: 1–3
Intensity: Moderate to high
Hold: 5–30 seconds

Starting position: Stand up straight, feet hip-width apart and weight distributed evenly on both feet. Put your arms at your sides and brace your abdominal muscles.

Movement: Place your right foot directly in front of your left foot, heel to toe, and squeeze your inner thighs together. Lift your arms out to your sides at shoulder level to help you balance. Hold. Return to the starting position, then repeat with your left foot in front. This completes one rep.

Tips and techniques:
- Pick a spot straight ahead of you to focus on.
- Contract your abdominal muscles, buttocks, and inner thighs to assist with balance.

Too hard? Hold on to the back of a chair or counter with one hand.

Too easy? Hold the position for 60 seconds.

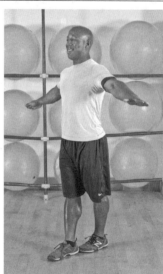

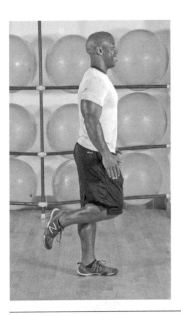

3 | Single-leg stance

Reps: 1
Sets: 1–3
Intensity: Moderate to high
Hold: 5–30 seconds

Starting position: Stand up straight, feet together and weight evenly distributed on both feet. Put your arms at your sides.

Movement: Lift your right foot a few inches off the floor, bending that knee slightly, and balance on your left leg. Hold. Lower your foot to the starting position, then repeat with your left leg. This completes one rep.

Tips and techniques:
- Pick a spot straight ahead to focus on.
- Maintain good posture throughout by keeping your chest lifted, your shoulders down and back, and your abdominal muscles braced.
- Breathe comfortably.

Too hard? Hold on to a chair or counter for support.

Too easy? Hold for 60 seconds, or close your eyes.

---

4 | Single-leg stance with side leg lift

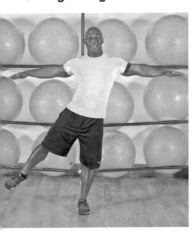

Reps: 1
Sets: 1–3
Intensity: High
Hold: 5–30 seconds

Starting position: Stand up straight, feet together and weight evenly distributed on both feet. Put your arms at your sides.

Movement: Lift your right foot out to the side a few inches off the floor, shifting your weight over to your left leg. Lift your arms out to each side at shoulder level to help you balance. Hold. Return to the starting position, then repeat with your left foot. This completes one rep.

Tips and techniques:
- Maintain good posture throughout by keeping your chest lifted, your shoulders down and back, and your abdominal muscles braced.
- Squeeze the buttock of the standing leg to help you balance.
- Breathe comfortably.

Too hard? Hold on to the back of a chair or counter with one hand.

Too easy? Hold for 60 seconds.

5 | Single-leg stance with back leg lift

Reps: 1
Sets: 1–3
Intensity: High
Hold: 5–30 seconds

Starting position: Stand up straight, feet together and weight evenly distributed on both feet. Put your arms at your sides.

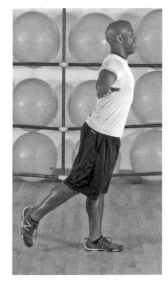

Movement: Lift your right foot straight behind you a few inches off the floor, shifting your weight over to your supporting leg. Lift your arms out to your sides at shoulder level to help you balance. Hold. Return to the starting position, then repeat with your left foot. This completes one rep.

Tips and techniques:
- Pick a spot straight ahead to focus on.
- Maintain good posture throughout by keeping your chest lifted, your shoulders down and back, and your abdominal muscles braced.
- Breathe comfortably.

Too hard? Hold on to the back of a chair or counter with one hand.

Too easy? Hold for 60 seconds.

6 | Single-leg stance with ankle circles

Reps: 1
Sets: 1–3
Intensity: High
Tempo: Go at your own pace

Starting position: Stand up straight with your feet together, arms at your sides, and weight evenly distributed on both feet.

Movement: Bend your right knee, lifting that leg up in front of you. Put both hands beneath the right thigh as you shift your weight over to the supporting leg. Slowly perform ankle circles with the raised ankle 10 times in each direction. Return to the starting position, then repeat with your left leg. This completes one rep.

Tips and techniques:
- Pick a spot straight ahead to focus on.
- Squeeze the buttock of the standing leg to help you balance.
- Breathe comfortably.

Too hard? Stand with your back against a wall, or sit in a chair to do the exercise.

Too easy? Hold the single-leg stance for 60 seconds while doing ankle circles.

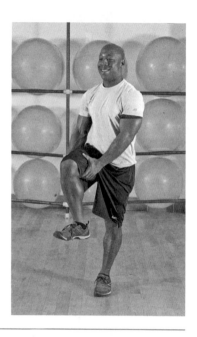

7 | Standing calf stretch

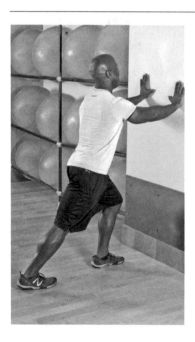

Reps: 3–4
Sets: 1
Intensity: Light
Hold: 10–30 seconds

Starting position: Stand up straight in front of a wall with your arms extended at shoulder height.

Movement: Place your hands on the wall. Extend your right leg straight back and press the heel toward the floor. Let your left leg bend as you do so. Hold. Return to the starting position, then repeat with your left leg. This completes one rep.

Tips and techniques:
- Stretch to the point of mild tension, not pain.
- Hold a full-body lean from the ankle as you stretch.
- Maintain neutral posture, with your shoulders down and back.

Too hard? Hold on to the back of a chair and do not press as far into the stretch.

Too easy? While holding on to the banister, balance on the front half of your feet at the edge of a stair. Your heels should extend into the air. Drop both heels until you feel the stretch in your calves.

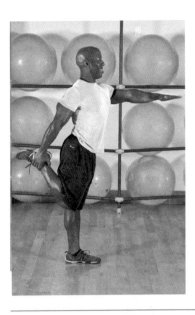

8 | Quadriceps stretch

Reps: 3–4
Sets: 1
Intensity: Moderate
Hold: 10–30 seconds

Starting position: Stand up straight, feet together and weight distributed evenly on both feet. Put your hands at your sides.

Movement: Bend your right knee and reach back with your right hand to grasp your foot and lift it toward your buttock. Raise your left arm to help you balance. Hold. Slowly lower your foot to the floor to return to the starting position, then repeat with your left leg. This completes one rep.

Tips and techniques:
- Stretch to the point of mild tension, not pain.
- Pull in your abdominal muscles and tighten the buttock of the supporting leg.
- Breathe comfortably.

Too hard? Place a yoga strap around your foot to assist with the stretch. Hold on to a chair for support if necessary.

Too easy? Press the hip of your supporting leg forward to increase the stretch.

9 | Alternating hamstring stretch

Reps: 3–4
Sets: 1
Intensity: Moderate to high
Hold: 10–30 seconds

Starting position: Lie on your back with both knees bent and feet flat on the floor.

Movement: Grasp your right leg with both hands behind the thigh. Extend your leg to lift your right foot toward the ceiling. Straighten the leg as much as possible without locking the knee and flex the ankle to stretch the calf muscles. Hold. Return to the starting position, then repeat with the left leg. This completes one rep.

Tips and techniques:
- Stretch to the point of mild tension, not pain. You should feel no pressure behind the knee.
- Relax your shoulders down and back into the floor.
- Breathe comfortably.

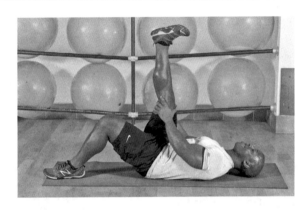

Too hard? Sit up straight in a chair. Extend your right leg straight out in front of you with the heel grounded on the floor and the toes pointing to the ceiling. Place your hands on top of your left thigh. Hinge forward from your hip while maintaining a neutral spine. Hold. Repeat with the left leg, placing your hands on your right thigh. This completes one rep.

Too easy? Stand upright and extend your right leg straight in front of you with your foot on a chair seat or counter. Flex your ankle. Place your hands on top of your right thigh. Hinge forward from the hip while maintaining a neutral spine. Repeat with the left leg. This completes one rep.

Balance in Motion Workout

Everyday acts—strolling down the street, walking up or down stairs, turning to look behind you—demand dynamic balance, the ability to anticipate and react to changes as you move. This workout hones that ability considerably, which helps prevent falls.

If you've had a hip replacement, ask your doctor if you need to modify any of the movements, particularly in exercise 2, "Braiding." Otherwise, focus on good form, rather than worrying about how many reps you can complete. If you find an exercise especially difficult, do fewer reps or try the easier variation. As you improve, try a harder variation. Before you start, be sure to read "Starting balance workouts safely," page 18.

Equipment: Sturdy chair (optional), counter (optional).

1 | Soccer kick

Reps: 10 on each side
Sets: 1–3
Intensity: Moderate
Tempo: 2–1–2

Starting position: Stand up straight with your feet together and your hands on your hips.

Movement: Point your right foot out to the right side and lift your arms out to the sides at shoulder level. Lift up your right foot and slowly sweep it diagonally in front of you as if kicking a soccer ball with the inside of your foot. Hold. Slowly bring your foot back to the right side. Finish all reps, then repeat with the left leg. This completes one set.

Tips and techniques:
- Keep your hips even and maintain neutral posture throughout.
- Tighten your abdominal muscles and squeeze the buttock of the standing leg.
- Breathe comfortably.

Too hard? Hold on to the back of a chair with one hand for support.

Too easy? Hold for four counts.

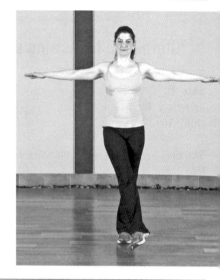

2 | Braiding

Reps: 10 right, 10 left
Sets: 1–3
Intensity: Light to moderate
Tempo: Slow and controlled

Starting position: Stand up straight, feet together and weight evenly distributed on both feet. Put your arms at your sides.

Movement: Step toward the right with your right foot. Cross over with your left foot, step out again with the right foot, and cross under with your left foot. Continue this braiding for 10 steps to the right, then bring your feet together. Hold until steady. Now do 10 steps of braiding to the left side of the room. This completes one set.

Tips and techniques:
- Maintain neutral posture throughout.
- Look ahead of you instead of down at your feet.
- Breathe comfortably.

Too hard? Hold on to a counter.

Too easy? Pick up your pace while staying in control of the movement.

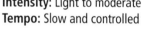
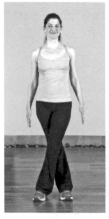
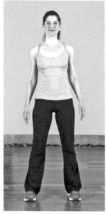
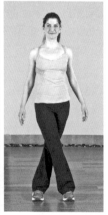

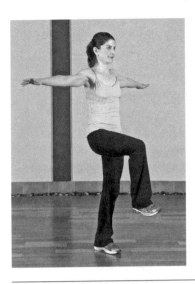

3 | Rock step

Reps: 10 on each side
Sets: 1–3
Intensity: Moderate to high
Tempo: 2–2–2

Starting position: Stand up straight, feet together and weight evenly distributed on both feet. Lift your arms out to each side.

Movement: Step forward with your right foot and lift up your left knee. Hold. Step back with your left foot and lift up your right knee. This is one rep. Finish all reps with the right foot leading, then repeat by leading with the left foot. This completes one set.

Tips and techniques:
- Tighten the buttock of the standing leg for stability.
- Maintain good posture throughout.
- Breathe comfortably.

Too hard? Hold on to the back of a chair with one hand for support.

Too easy? Hold the knee up for a count of four.

4 | Side squat with knee lift and rotation

Reps: 10 per side
Sets: 1–3
Intensity: Moderate
Tempo: 2–2

Starting position: Stand up straight with your feet together and your arms at your sides.

Movement: Step out to the right, hinge at your hips, and bend your knees

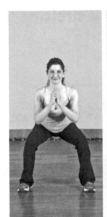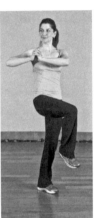

to lower your buttocks into a squat as if sitting in a chair. Simultaneously, clasp your hands loosely in front of your chest. Exhaling as you lift your body out of the squat, bring your right foot toward your left knee as you rotate your upper body to the right. Return to the squat. This is one rep. Finish all reps, then repeat the sequence stepping out to the left. This completes one set.

Tips and techniques:
- Keep your spine neutral and your shoulders down and back.
- Keep your knees aligned over your ankles and pointing forward as you squat.
- Your knees should extend no farther than the tips of your toes.

Too hard? Make the squat smaller.

Too easy? Hold the squat for four counts.

5 | Curtsies

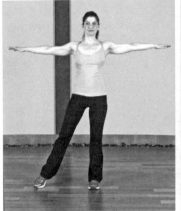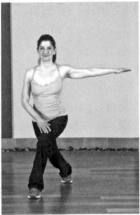

Reps: 10 on each side
Sets: 1–3
Intensity: Moderate to high
Tempo: 2–2

Starting position: Stand up straight with your right leg out to your side, toe touching the floor. Extend your arms to each side at shoulder level.

Movement: Bring your right foot behind your left leg, place your weight on the ball of the rear foot, and bend your knees as if curtseying. Touch your right hand to your left knee. Exhale as you return to the starting position. Finish all reps, then repeat with your left leg. This completes one set.

Tips and techniques:
- Keep your spine neutral and your shoulders down and back.
- When returning to the starting position, exhale and tighten the buttock of your front leg as you lift up to help you balance.

Too hard? Do fewer reps.

Too easy? As you rise up from the curtsey, lift your leg out to the side in the air, then return to the curtsey.

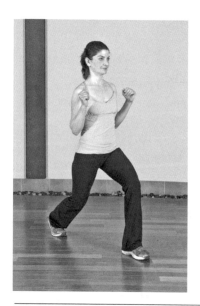

6 | Reverse lunge

Reps: 10 on each side
Sets: 1–3
Intensity: Moderate to high
Tempo: 2–2

Starting position: Stand up straight, feet together and weight evenly distributed on both feet. Put your arms at your sides.

Movement: Step back on the ball of your right foot and sink into a lunge by bending your knees so that your left knee aligns with your left ankle and your right knee points to the floor. Simultaneously, bring your hands up in front of your chest, elbows bent. Exhale as you return to the starting position. Finish all reps, then repeat stepping back on your left foot. This completes one set.

Tips and techniques:

- Keep your weight evenly distributed between the right and left foot.
- In the lunge position, your shoulder, hip, and rear knee should be aligned.
- Keep your spine neutral and your shoulders down and back.

Too hard? Make the lunge smaller.

Too easy? Hold the lunge for four counts before returning to the starting position.

7 | Chest stretch

Reps: 3–4
Sets: 1
Intensity: Light
Hold: 10–30 seconds

Starting position: Stand in a doorway facing forward. Extend your right arm and put your right hand on the edge of the door frame slightly below shoulder level, palm forward. Keep your shoulders down and back.

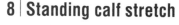

Movement: Slowly turn your body to the left, away from the part of the door frame that you're touching, until you feel the stretch in your chest and shoulder. Hold. Return to the starting position, then switch arm positions and repeat with your left hand on the door frame. This completes one rep.

Tips and techniques:

- Stretch to the point of mild tension, not pain.
- Breathe comfortably.

Too hard? Place your hand a bit lower on the door frame and don't turn as far.

Too easy? Lift your hand a bit higher on the door frame, without going above shoulder level, to increase the stretch.

8 | Standing calf stretch

Reps: 3–4
Sets: 1
Intensity: Light
Hold: 10–30 seconds

Starting position: Stand up straight in front of a wall with arms extended.

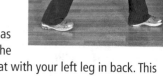

Movement: Place your hands on the wall with fingers at shoulder level. Extend your right leg straight back and press the heel toward the floor. Let your left leg bend as you do so. Hold. Return to the starting position, then repeat with your left leg in back. This completes one rep.

Tips and techniques:

- Stretch to the point of mild tension, not pain.
- Hold a full-body lean from the ankle as you stretch.
- Maintain neutral posture with your shoulders down and back.

Too hard? Hold on to the back of a chair and do not press as far into the stretch.

Too easy? While holding on to the banister, balance on the front half of your feet at the edge of a stair. Your heels should extend into the air. Drop both heels until you feel the stretch in your calves.

Balance 360 Workout

A hard, flat surface like a floor makes it easier to maintain balance. Introducing instability by standing on a surface that is squishy or easy to tip bumps up the challenge for balance exercises. This workout uses a piece of equipment called the Step360, which is a flat, nonslip platform on top of two inflatable rings. To remain balanced, you'll need to engage a wider-than-usual range of muscles, including your core muscles.

It helps to practice these exercises a few times on the floor before moving to the Step360. Focus on good form, holding a position steadily, and moving smoothly through each exercise, rather than worrying about how many reps you can complete. If you find an exercise especially difficult, do fewer reps or try the easier variation. As you improve, try a harder variation. Before you start, be sure to read "Starting balance workouts safely," page 18.

Equipment: Step360.

1 | Standing knee lifts

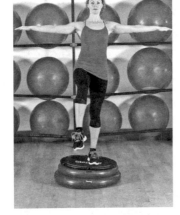

Reps: 10 on each side
Sets: 1–3
Intensity: Moderate
Tempo: 2–2

Starting position: Stand up straight on the center of the Step360, feet together and weight evenly distributed on both feet. Put your arms out to each side at shoulder level.

Movement: Lift your right knee up toward the ceiling as high as is comfortable, then lower your foot to the step. Finish all reps, then repeat with the left leg. This completes one set.

Tips and techniques:
- Squeeze the buttock of the standing leg to help you balance.
- Brace your abdominal muscles throughout the movement.
- Keep your chest lifted and your shoulders down and back.

Too hard? Don't lift up your knee as high.

Too easy? Lower and raise your knee without letting your foot touch the step.

2 | Side squat with back leg lift

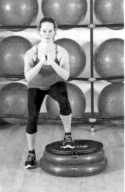

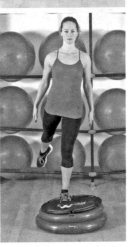

Reps: 10 on each side
Sets: 1–3
Intensity: Moderate
Tempo: 2–2

Starting position: Stand up straight on the Step360, slightly to the right of its center, with feet together and weight evenly distributed on both feet. Put your arms at your sides.

Movement: Step to the right off the Step360, hinge forward at your hips, and bend your knees to lower your buttocks into a squat as if sitting down in a chair. Simultaneously clasp your hands loosely in front of your chest. Balance your weight evenly with your right foot on the floor and your left foot on the Step360. Lift up from the squat, extending your right foot back in the air and bringing your arms to your sides, then return to the squat. Finish all reps, then repeat, stepping off with the left leg. This completes one set.

Tips and techniques:
- Keep your spine neutral and your shoulders down and back.
- Keep your knees aligned over your ankles and pointing forward as you squat.
- Squeeze the buttock of the standing leg as you lift up from the squat to help you balance.

Too hard? Do the exercise on the floor.

Too easy? Hold the lift for four counts before finishing the movement.

3 | Rock step

Reps: 10 on each side
Sets: 1–3

Intensity: Moderate to high
Tempo: 2–2–2

Starting position: Stand up straight on the floor behind the Step360, feet together and weight evenly distributed on both feet. Put your arms at your sides.

Movement: Step forward with your right foot onto the center of the Step360 and lift your left knee toward the ceiling. Put your arms out to each side, elbows slightly bent, to help you balance. Hold. Step back down off the Step360 onto the floor with your left foot and lift your right knee. This is one rep. Finish all reps with the right foot leading, then repeat, leading with the left foot. This completes one set.

Tips and techniques:

- Pick a spot straight ahead to focus on.
- Maintain neutral posture throughout the movement.

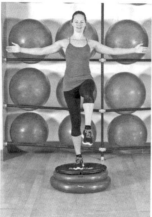 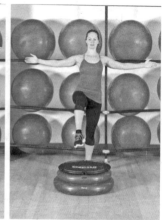

- Squeeze the buttock of the standing leg as you lift up to help you balance.

Too hard? Do the exercise on the floor.

Too easy? Hold the knee lift for four counts instead of two.

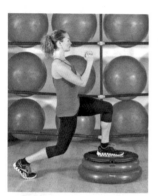

4 | Reverse lunges

Reps: 10 on each side
Sets: 1–3
Intensity: Moderate to high
Tempo: 2–2

Starting position: Stand up straight on the center of the Step360, feet together and weight evenly distributed on both feet. Put your arms at your sides.

Movement: Step back off the Step360 onto the floor on the ball of your right foot and sink into a lunge with your left knee aligned over your left ankle and right knee pointing to the floor. Simultaneously, bring your hands up in front of your chest, elbows bent. Exhale as you return to the starting position on top of the Step360. Finish all reps, then repeat with your left leg in back. This completes one set.

Tips and techniques:

- Position yourself on the Step360 so that you can complete the backward lunge with ease without brushing the edge with your rear knee.
- In the lunge position, your shoulder, hip, and rear knee should be aligned.
- Squeeze the buttock of the standing leg as you lift back up onto the Step360 to help you balance.

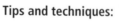

Too hard? Do the exercise on the floor.

Too easy? Hold the lunge for four counts before returning to the starting position.

5 | Squat with knee lift

Reps: 10 on each side
Sets: 1-3
Intensity: Moderate to high
Tempo: 2-2-2

Starting position: Stand up straight on the Step360, feet hip-width apart and weight evenly distributed on both feet. Put your hands at your sides.

Movement: Hinge forward at your hips and bend your knees to lower your buttocks toward the floor as if sitting down in a chair, stopping with your buttocks above knee level. Simultaneously, clasp your hands loosely in front of your chest. Rise up from the squat, lifting your right knee up toward the ceiling and extending your arms out to the sides. Lower your right foot back into the starting position. Finish all reps, then repeat with your left leg. This completes one set.

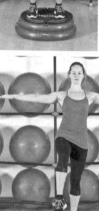

Tips and techniques:

- Keep your hips, knees, and toes all pointing forward.
- Brace your abdominal muscles throughout the movement.
- Squeeze the buttock of the standing leg to help you balance as you rise up from the squat and do the knee lift.

Too hard? Do the exercise on the floor.

Too easy? Hold the knee lift for four counts.

6 | Alternating kneeling opposite arm and leg raise

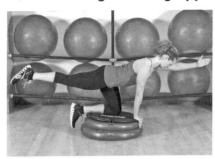

Reps: 10
Sets: 1–3
Rest: 30–90 seconds between sets
Intensity: Moderate to high
Tempo: 2–4–2

Starting position: Kneel on all fours on the Step360 with your hands and knees directly aligned under your shoulders and hips. Keep your head and spine neutral.

Movement: Extend your right leg off the Step360 behind you while reaching out in front of you with your left arm, thumb up. Keeping your hips and shoulders squared, try to bring the leg and arm parallel to the floor. Hold. Return to the starting position, then repeat with your left leg and right arm. This completes one rep.

Tips and techniques:
- Brace your abdominal muscles during the exercise.
- Imagine someone pulling your arm and leg to lengthen your torso.
- Keep your head and neck neutral.

Too hard? Extend your right arm; return to the starting position. Extend your left leg; return to the starting position. Repeat with the left arm, followed by the right leg. This completes one rep.

Too easy? Move your extended arm and leg on a diagonal (think of a clock: instead of noon and six, move them to one and seven or 11 and five, depending on which arm and leg is in action).

7 | Kneeling torso rotation

Reps: 3–4 per side
Sets: 1
Intensity: Light to moderate
Tempo: 2–2–2

Starting position: Kneel with your knees a few inches apart on the Step360. Place your right hand on the Step360 directly under your shoulder. Touch the back of your head gently with your left hand.

Movement: Rotating your torso down to the right, bring your left elbow down to your right wrist. Exhale and slowly rotate up to the left, lifting your left elbow up so it points toward the ceiling as high as you can go. Hold. Finish all reps, then repeat on the other side.

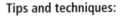

Tips and techniques:
- Follow your elbow with your eyes throughout the movement.
- Try to keep your weight evenly distributed on both knees.
- Breathe comfortably.

Too hard? Do the exercise on the floor.

Too easy? Hold for four counts with the elbow pointing toward the ceiling.

8 | Standing hamstring stretch

Reps: 3–4
Sets: 1
Intensity: Light to moderate
Hold: 10–30 seconds

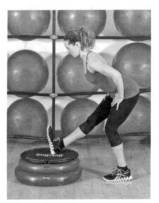

Starting position: Stand up straight on the floor behind the Step360. Extend your right leg in front of you so that your right heel rests on top of the Step360.

Movement: Straighten your right leg as much as possible without locking your knee. As you do so, flex the ankle to stretch the calf muscles. Place your hands on your upper thighs, then hinge forward from the hips and bend your left knee slightly. You should feel mild tension in your right hamstring and no pressure behind that knee. Hold. Return to the starting position, then repeat with the left leg. This is one rep.

Tips and techniques:
- Stretch to the point of mild tension, not pain.
- Keep your hips and shoulders squared.
- Squeeze the buttock of the standing leg to help you balance.

Too hard? Do the exercise on the floor.

Too easy? Hinge farther forward to increase the stretch.

Balance on the Beam Workout

This workout steps up the challenge with three elements. The soft surface of the Beamfit Beam introduces instability. The raised height—a mere two inches—puts your feet at different levels in certain exercises, much as you would encounter when stepping off a curb. Keeping your feet on the six-inch-wide beam during other exercises makes balancing more difficult. Mastering this workout will do a great deal to enhance your balance. Warning: If you are older and have walking problems, a strip of masking tape on the floor will be a safer substitute for the balance beam.

You may do this workout barefoot or wearing sneakers. Focus on good form, rather than worrying about how many reps you can complete. If you find an exercise especially difficult, do fewer reps or try the easier variation. As you improve, try a harder variation. Before you start, be sure to read "Starting balance workouts safely," page 18.

Equipment: Beamfit Beam, masking tape (optional).

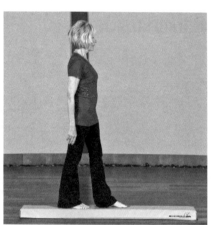

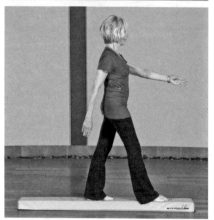

1 | Mambo step

Reps: 10 on each side
Sets: 1–3
Intensity: Light to moderate
Tempo: 2–2

Starting position: Stand up straight at the center of the balance beam. Position your left foot about four inches ahead of your right foot. Put your arms at your side.

Movement: During the mambo, you rock one foot forward and back. Using this mambo rhythm, slowly bring your right foot forward ahead of the left foot, press down momentarily on the beam, then slowly bring your right foot back to the starting position. As you do the step, let your arms swing comfortably slightly backward and forward as a counterbalance. Stepping forward and backward this way, finish all reps, then repeat the sequence starting with your right foot in front. This completes one set.

Tips and techniques:

- Squeeze your inner thighs to help you balance.
- Pick a spot straight ahead to focus on.
- Brace your abdominal muscles throughout the movement.

Too hard? Do the exercise on the floor.

Too easy? Instead of doing the mambo step, try swinging your rear foot forward and then backward in the air without touching the balance beam. Finish all reps, then repeat with the other foot.

2 | Tandem stand with rotation

Reps: 1 on each side
Sets: 1–3
Intensity: Moderate to high
Tempo: 2–2–2

Starting position: Stand up straight at the center of the balance beam with your right foot positioned directly in front of your left foot, heel to toe. Put your arms at your sides.

Movement: Bring your arms out to each side at shoulder level. Slowly rotate your head and torso toward the left side of the room. Hold. Slowly return to the starting position. This is one rep. Now repeat the sequence with your left foot forward, rotating your head and torso to the right side of the room. This completes one set.

Tips and techniques:
- Squeeze your inner thighs together to help you balance.
- Keep your weight evenly distributed on both feet.
- Brace your abdominal muscles throughout the movement.

_____

Too hard? Do the exercise on the floor.

Too easy? Hold the rotation for four counts.

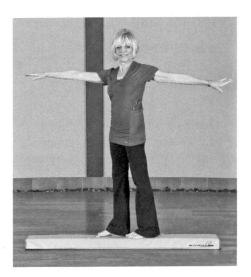

3 | Walk forward, walk back

Reps: 10 on each side
Sets: 1–3
Intensity: Moderate
Tempo: 2–2

Starting position: Stand up straight near one end of the balance beam. Position your right foot in front of your left foot. Put your arms at your sides.

Movement: Lift your arms out to each side at shoulder level. Step forward several inches on the beam with your right foot, then slide your left foot forward to the heel of your right foot. Step forward again with your right foot, then slide your left foot forward. Step backward several inches on the beam with your left foot, then slide your right foot backward to the toes of your left foot. Step backward again with your left foot, then slide your right foot backward. This is one rep. Finish all reps, then repeat with your left foot forward. This completes one set.

Tips and techniques:
- Brace your abdominal muscles throughout the movement.
- As you bring your feet together, squeeze your inner thighs together to help you balance.
- Maintain neutral posture.

_____

Too hard? Do the exercise on the floor.

Too easy? Step forward, slide forward, step forward, slide forward, lift the knee of the front leg toward the ceiling, and then put that foot back on the beam. Step backward, slide backward, step backward, slide backward, lift the knee of the front leg toward the ceiling, and then put that foot back on the beam. Finish all reps, then repeat with the other leg forward.

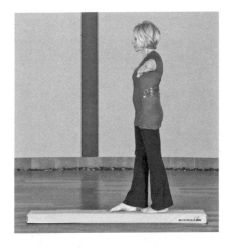

4 | Rock step with knee lifts

Reps: 10 on each side
Sets: 1–3
Intensity: High
Tempo: 2–2

Starting position: Stand up straight near the center of the balance beam. Position your right foot in front of your left foot and put your arms out to each side at shoulder level.

Movement: Slowly step forward on the beam with your right foot and lift your left knee toward the ceiling. Step backward onto the center of the beam behind you with your left foot and lift your right knee toward the ceiling. This is one rep. Finish all reps, then repeat with your left foot forward. This completes one set.

Tips and techniques:

- Maintain neutral posture.
- Always step in the center of the beam.
- Brace your abdominal muscles throughout the movement and squeeze the buttock of the standing leg to help you balance.

Too hard? Do the exercise on the floor.

Too easy? Hold knee lifts for two counts.

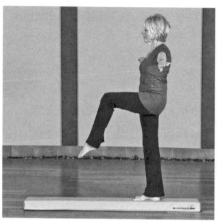
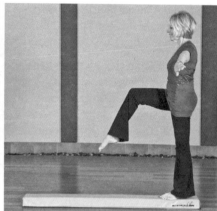

5 | Stationary lunges

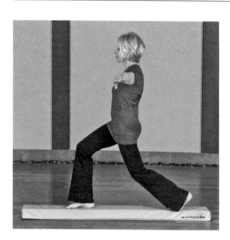

Reps: 10 on each side
Sets: 1–3
Intensity: High
Tempo: 2–2

Starting position: Stand up straight near the front of the beam with your right foot in front of your left foot. Step way back on the ball of your left foot and sink a few inches into a lunge by bending both knees several inches so that your right knee aligns over your right ankle and your left knee points to the beam. Lift your hands out to your sides at shoulder level to help with balance.

Movement: Slowly lower your left knee down toward the beam, then lift back up to the starting position. Finish all reps, then repeat with your left foot in front.

Tips and techniques:

- Brace your abdominal muscles throughout the movement.
- Maintain neutral posture.
- Exhale as you lift up from the lunge position.

Too hard? Do the exercise on the floor.

Too easy? Hold the lunge for four counts.

6 | Side squat, forward lunge

Reps: 10 on each side
Sets: 1–3
Intensity: Moderate to high
Tempo: 2–2–2–2

Starting position: Stand up straight at the center of the balance beam. Position your right foot a few inches ahead of your left foot and raise your arms to the side at shoulder level.

Movement: This four-part movement is side squat, lunge, side squat, stand, then repeat. First, step to the left of the balance beam with your left foot, hinging forward at your hips and bending your knees into a squat as if sitting down in a chair, while clasping your hands loosely in front of your chest with elbows bent. Second, lift up from the squat, bring your left foot to the front of the balance beam, and sink into a small lunge by bending both knees so that the left knee aligns over your left ankle and the right knee points to the beam. Let your right arm swing forward and your left arm swing slightly backward as a counterbalance. Third, lift up from the lunge and return to the side squat position with hands clasped loosely in front of your chest. Fourth, lift up once more from the squat and bring your feet back to the starting position, right foot a few inches ahead of left foot, as you raise your arms out to each side at shoulder level. This is one rep. Finish all reps, then repeat with your left foot forward so that the squat is to the right side.

Tips and techniques:

- Brace your abdominal muscles and maintain neutral posture throughout the movement.
- Squeeze the buttock of the leg on the beam to help you balance.
- Exhale on the lift off the floor.

Too hard? Do the exercise on the floor.

Too easy? Hold lunge for four counts instead of two.

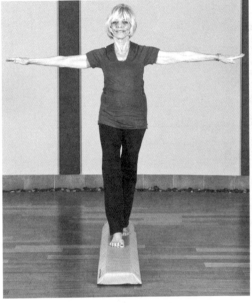
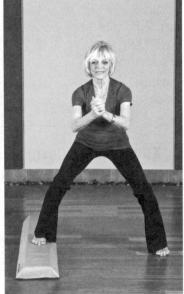

7 | Standing calf stretch

Reps: 3–4
Sets: 1
Intensity: Light to moderate
Hold: 10–30 seconds

Starting position: Stand up straight on the floor, facing the beam with your arms at your sides. Step onto the top of the beam on the front half of both feet, allowing your heels to extend past the edge of the beam.

Movement: Slowly press your heels down toward the floor, keeping your toes on top of the beam. Lift your arms out to each side to help you balance. Hold. Return to starting position. This is one rep.

Tips and techniques:

- Stretch to the point of mild tension, not pain.
- Hold a full-body lean from the ankle as you stretch.
- Maintain neutral posture with your shoulders down and back.

Too hard? Do not press as far into the stretch.

Too easy? Lean farther forward into the stretch.

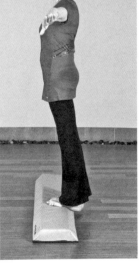
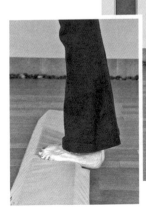

8 | Pretzel stretch

Reps: 3–4
Sets: 1
Intensity: Moderate
Hold: 10–30 seconds

Starting position: Lie on your back on top of the balance beam, with your right knee bent and that foot in the center of the beam. Rest your left ankle on your right kneecap. Your left knee should point toward the wall.

Movement: Relax your shoulders down and back as you lift your right foot off the beam, grasping the back of your right thigh with both hands, until you feel tightness in your left hip and buttock. Hold. Return to the starting position. Repeat on the other side. This is one rep.

Tips and techniques:

- Stretch to the point of mild tension, not pain.
- Hold as still as possible without bouncing.
- Breathe comfortably.

Too hard? Lie on your back with your knees bent and both feet on the beam. Cross your right knee over your left. Holding your right knee, gently bring your both knees toward your chest. Repeat on the other side. This is one rep.

Too easy? Extend the leg you are holding toward the ceiling.

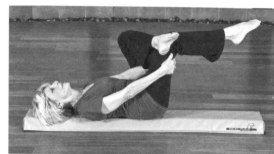

9 | Kneeling hip flexor stretch

Reps: 3–4
Sets: 1
Intensity: Moderate
Hold: 10–30 seconds

Starting position: Kneel with your right knee on the balance beam and left foot on the floor with the knee bent at a 90-degree angle. You may place your hands on your left thigh for support.

Movement: Lean forward, pressing into the hip of your right leg while keeping your left foot on the floor. Hold. Repeat on the other side. This completes one rep.

Tips and techniques:

- Stretch to the point of mild tension, not pain.
- Maintain a neutral spine while keeping hips and shoulders even.
- Keep your shoulders down and back and brace your abdominal muscles.

Too hard? Lie on your back on the beam. Pull your right knee toward your chest and extend your left leg on the floor next to the beam. Flex your left ankle and press your calf down toward the floor. You will feel this stretch in front of the extended leg, and in the lower back and buttock of the bent knee. Hold. Repeat on the other side. This completes one rep.

Too easy? As you lean forward, pressing into the hip of your right leg, lift your right arm up and curve it over your head to increase the stretch.

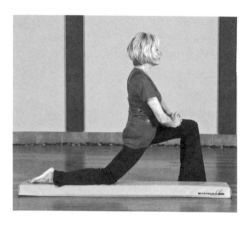

Yoga Balance Workout

Yoga does an excellent job of strengthening and stretching muscles essential for balance. The yoga poses described below challenge static balance, the ability to stand in one spot without swaying, and dynamic balance, the ability to anticipate and react to changes as you move. Successfully managing these tasks requires you to keep your center of gravity poised over a base of support. Focus on good form, rather than worrying about how many reps you can complete. If you find an exercise especially difficult, do fewer reps or try the easier variation. As you improve, try a harder variation. Before you start, be sure to read "Starting balance workouts safely," page 18.

Equipment: Mat, pillow (optional).

Yoga breathing

Yoga breathing, or pranayama, is relaxing and meditative. Try this simple technique while performing yoga poses, or do it for a few minutes once or twice during the day.

Lie on a mat with your feet on the floor, hip-width apart, and knees gently touching. Rest one hand on your heart and the other below your navel. Inhale and exhale through your nose, if possible (if not, breathe in through the nose, and out through softly parted lips). As you exhale, try to make a whispering sound at the back of your throat.

Start by tuning in to the way you breathe by inhaling and exhaling naturally for a few minutes. Notice how the air feels as it enters and exits your nostrils.

As you continue, begin counting silently forward (one, two, three …), then backward (…three, two, one). Gradually lengthen your breaths until each exhalation is twice as long as each inhalation. As you fill your lungs, feel your rib cage expand to the side and your lower belly rise and fall slightly. Focus on breathing slowly and smoothly.

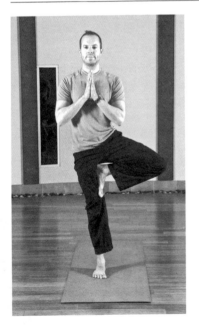

1 | Tree pose

Reps: 2–4
Sets: 1
Intensity: Moderate to high
Hold: 10 breaths or 10–30 seconds

Starting position: Stand up straight, feet hip-width apart and weight evenly distributed on both feet. Put your arms at your sides.

Movement: Slowly shift your weight to your right leg. Lift up your left foot and place it on the inside of your right leg above or below the knee. To help you balance, place the sole of your left foot firmly against your right leg and press your right leg against your left foot, grounding down through the standing leg for stability. Brace your abdominal muscles as you bend your elbows and bring your hands up in front of your chest in a prayer position. Hold. Return to the starting position, then repeat standing on your left leg.

This completes one rep.

Tips and techniques:
- Pick a spot straight ahead to focus on.
- Maintain neutral posture.
- Squeeze the buttock of the standing leg to help you balance.

Too hard? Place your left foot at your calf or ankle.

Too easy? Lift your foot higher on the supporting leg so that the heel is near your groin.

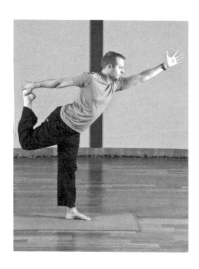

2 | Dancer

Reps: 2–4
Sets: 1
Intensity: Moderate to high
Hold: 5 breaths or 5–15 seconds

Starting position: Stand up straight, feet together and weight evenly distributed on both feet. Put your arms at your sides.

Movement: Raise your left arm forward at shoulder level, thumb up. Bend your right knee and reach back with your right hand to grasp your ankle or your foot and lift it toward your buttock. Align your knees. Inhale and lift your left arm higher to help you bal-ance. Hold. Return to the starting position, then repeat bending your left leg. This completes one rep.

Tips and techniques:
- Pick a spot straight ahead to focus on.
- Brace your abdominal muscles and squeeze the buttock of the standing leg.

Too hard? Instead of raising your arm, hold on to a sturdy chair or put one hand against the wall.

Too easy? Hold for 30–60 seconds.

3 | Crescent warrior

Reps: 2–4
Sets: 1
Intensity: Moderate to high
Hold: 5 breaths or 5–15 seconds

Starting position: Stand up straight, feet together and weight evenly distributed on both feet. Put your arms at your sides.

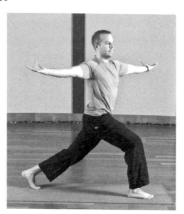

Movement: Place your hands on your right thigh as you step back onto the ball of your left foot and sink into a high lunge by bending your right knee so that it is aligned over the ankle. Keep your left leg straight and your head, shoulders, hips, and feet facing forward. Bring your hands out to each side at shoulder level, palms up. Slowly exhale and rotate your torso to the right, keeping your chin centered above your chest. Hold. Return to the starting position, then repeat by stepping back onto the ball of your right foot and rotating your torso toward the left.

Tips and techniques:
- Brace your abdominal muscles throughout.
- Try to keep your weight evenly distributed between both feet.
- Breathe comfortably or perform yoga breathing.

Too hard? Skip the rotation.

Too easy? Hold for 15–30 seconds.

4 | Warrior III

Reps: 2–4 per side
Sets: 1
Intensity: Moderate to high
Hold: 5 breaths or 5–15 seconds

Starting position: Stand up straight, feet together and weight

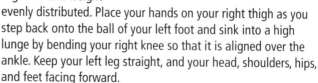

evenly distributed. Place your hands on your right thigh as you step back onto the ball of your left foot and sink into a high lunge by bending your right knee so that it is aligned over the ankle. Keep your left leg straight, and your head, shoulders, hips, and feet facing forward.

Movement: Shift your weight forward over your right leg. Simultaneously lift both arms forward in line with your shoulders, palms inward, and lift your left leg until it is parallel to the floor, flexing the ankle so that your toes point toward the floor. Your head, shoulders, and hips should be even and parallel to the floor. Hold. Exhale and return to the starting position. Finish all reps. Repeat the full sequence with your weight on your left leg.

Tips and techniques:
- Brace your abdominal muscles and squeeze the buttock of the supporting leg to help you balance.
- Think of someone pulling your arms forward and drawing your extended leg backward.
- Keep your head and spine neutral and your shoulders down.

Too hard? Slightly bend the knee of your supporting leg and do not lift your back leg as high.

Too easy? As you raise your back leg, reach your arms back alongside your body, palms toward the floor.

5 | Side plank

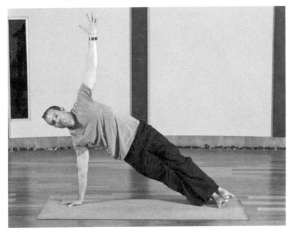

Reps: 2–4 per side
Sets: 1
Intensity: Moderate to high
Hold: 10 breaths or 10–30 seconds

Starting position: Kneel on all fours with your hands and knees directly aligned under your shoulders and hips. Extend both legs, hip-distance apart, feet flexed and toes touching the floor so that you balance your body in a line like a plank.

Movement: Roll to the outer edge of your right foot, stacking your left foot on top of the right. Raise your left arm up toward the ceiling, palm forward with fingers extended and wrist aligned directly over your shoulder. Brace your abdominal muscles. Keeping your shoulders, hips, and feet in a straight line, balance on your right hand. Hold. Return to the starting position. Finish all reps, then repeat on your left side.

Tips and techniques:

- Keep your head and spine neutral, and directly align your shoulder over the hand on the floor.
- Focus on lifting your bottom hip.
- Keep your shoulders down and back.

Too hard? To help you balance in the right side plank, bend your left knee and place your left foot on the floor in front of your right leg, toes pointing toward the wall in front of you.

Too easy? Lift your top foot up toward the ceiling.

6 | Figure four

Reps: 1 on each side
Sets: 1
Intensity: Moderate
Hold: 5 breaths or 5–15 seconds

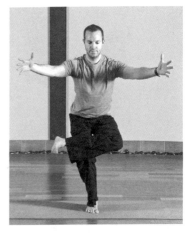

Starting position: Stand up straight, feet hip-width apart, and weight evenly distributed on both feet. Put your arms at your sides.

Movement: Standing on your right foot, bend your left knee and place your flexed left ankle above your right knee in a figure-four position. To help you balance, press your left ankle firmly against your right leg and squeeze your right leg against your left ankle. Bring your arms to shoulder level, elbows slightly bent and palms inward.

Now, extend your hips backward as if sitting down in a chair, while moving your arms forward to a wide V-position. Brace your abdominal muscles. Hold. Return to the starting position. Repeat the sequence standing on your left foot.

Tips and techniques:

- Exhale as you sink into the pose.
- Draw your shoulders down away from your ears.
- Breathe comfortably or practice yoga breathing.

Too hard? Put your hand against the wall for support.

Too easy? Hold for 10 breaths or 10–30 seconds.

7 | Upward-facing dog

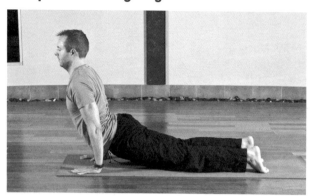

Reps: 2–4
Sets: 1
Intensity: Moderate
Hold: 5 breaths or 5–15 seconds

Starting position: Lie on your stomach with your hands under your shoulders, elbows close to your sides. Extend your legs comfortably and press the tops of your feet against the floor.

Movement: Inhale, pushing with your hands and feet simultaneously to lift your upper torso and hips off the floor. Keep your chin parallel to the floor as you try to fully straighten your arms without locking your elbows. Hold. Return to the starting position.

Tips and techniques:

- Lift upward only to the point of mild tension, not pain.
- Do not lock your elbows when fully straightening your arms.
- Breathe comfortably or practice yoga breathing.

Too hard? Do not lift upward as far.

Too easy? Hold the lift for 10 breaths or 10–30 seconds.

8 | Downward-facing dog

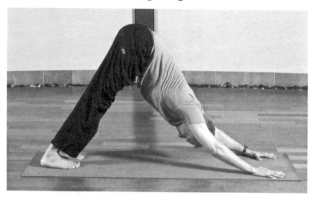

Reps: 2–4
Sets: 1
Intensity: Light to moderate
Hold: 10 breaths or 10–30 seconds

Starting position: Start on your hands and knees with your fingers extended.

Movement: Exhale as you lift your knees off the floor, straightening your legs without locking the knees until you are in an upside-down V. While maintaining a neutral neck and spine, align your ears with your biceps. Try to keep your weight evenly distributed between your hands and feet. Press your heels down toward the floor, if possible, while keeping your shoulders rolled back. Hold. Return to the starting position.

Tips and techniques:

- Keep your shoulders rolled back as you lengthen your spine.
- Brace your abdominal muscles throughout.
- Breathe comfortably or practice yoga breathing.

Too hard? Bend your knees slightly and let your heels come up off the floor.

Too easy? Hold 30–60 seconds.

Note: Special thanks to the Equinox fitness club at 131 Dartmouth Street in Boston for the use of its facilities, and to the following Equinox personal trainers, instructors, and staff members for demonstrating the exercises depicted in this report: Kristy DiScipio, Josie Gardiner, Ian Lemieux, Joy Prouty, Cynthia Roth, and RaShaun Smith.

Resources

Organizations

American Academy of Otolaryngology—Head and Neck Surgery
1650 Diagonal Road
Alexandria, VA 22314
703-836-4444
www.entnet.org

This is a national professional organization for specialists called ENTs who treat problems of the ear, nose, and throat or related structures. Its website offers health information and a referral service to locate ENTs.

American College of Sports Medicine
401 W. Michigan St.
Indianapolis, IN 46202
317-637-9200
www.acsm.org

ACSM educates and certifies fitness professionals, such as personal trainers, and funds research on exercise. A referral service on the website locates ASCM-certified personal trainers.

American Council on Exercise
4851 Paramount Drive
San Diego, CA 92123
888-825-3636 (toll-free)
www.acefitness.org

ACE is a nonprofit organization that promotes fitness. Its website offers a library of free exercise videos and a referral service to locate ACE-certified personal trainers.

American Physical Therapy Association
1111 N. Fairfax St.
Alexandria, VA 22314
800-999-2782 (toll-free)
www.apta.org

This national professional organization fosters advances in physical therapy education, research, and practice. A referral system on the website locates board-certified clinical specialists with additional training in specific areas.

Arthritis Foundation
1330 Peachtree St., Suite 100
Atlanta, GA 30309
800-283-7800 (toll-free)
www.arthritis.org

This national nonprofit organization has local chapters in many states. The website offers educational materials on arthritis, pain control, treatments, alternative therapies, and more. Local chapters may offer classes, such as Walk with Ease, a six-week, instructor-led walking program designed for people with arthritis. (Alternatively, you can buy the *Walk with Ease* book from the foundation's website.)

National Institute on Aging
Building 31, Room 5C27
31 Center Drive, MSC 2292
Bethesda, MD 20892
800-222-2225 (toll-free)
www.nia.nih.gov
www.nia.nih.gov/Go4Life

The National Institute on Aging has a free, easy-to-follow booklet and companion video packed with good exercises called *Exercise & Physical Activity*. The NIA's Go4Life website hosts an exercise campaign aimed at enhancing endurance, strength, balance, and flexibility for people ages 50 and older, including those recovering from injuries or living with chronic illnesses.

Special Health Reports

The following Special Health Reports from Harvard Medical School may also help you improve your balance. These reports can be ordered by calling 877-649-9457 (toll-free) or online at www.health.harvard.edu.

Core Exercises: 6 Workouts to Tighten Your Abs, Strengthen Your Back, and Improve Balance
Edward M. Phillips, M.D., Josie Gardiner, and Joy Prouty
(Harvard Medical School, 2013)

Your core—which includes back, side, pelvic, and buttock muscles—forms a sturdy central link between your upper body and lower body. Core muscles need to be strong, yet flexible. These workouts help build core strength.

Gentle Core Exercises: Start Toning Your Abs, Building Your Back Muscles, and Reclaiming Core Fitness Today
Edward M. Phillips, M.D., and Josie Gardiner
(Harvard Medical School, 2013)

A strong core can contribute to balance and stability, while helping maintain a healthy back and good posture. This special program of gentle core exercises and stretches complements the *Core Exercises* report (above), which contains harder exercises.

The Joint Pain Relief Workout: Healing Exercises for Your Shoulders, Hips, Knees, and Ankles
Edward M. Phillips, M.D., Josie Gardiner, and Joy Prouty
(Harvard Medical School, 2014)

The right set of exercises can be a long-lasting way to tame ankle, knee, hip, or shoulder pain. The workouts in this report may help you postpone, or avoid, surgery on a problem joint.

Strength and Power Training: A Guide for Older Adults
Julie K. Silver, M.D.
(Harvard Medical School, 2013)

A guide to easy strength-training exercises, plus adaptations to help build power—a combination of strength and speed.

Workout Workbook: 9 Complete Workouts to Help You Get Fit and Healthy
Edward M. Phillips, M.D., Josie Gardiner, and Joy Prouty
(Harvard Medical School, 2013)

Nine workouts to try at home, take on the road, or mix into your gym routine. Core, strength, stability ball, power challenge, travel, and other workouts help you enhance fitness.

Glossary

arrhythmia: A hindrance in the speed or rhythm of the heartbeat that may interfere with blood supply to the brain, spurring sudden weakness, lightheadedness, or dizziness that affect balance, or more serious problems like fainting or a heart attack.

balance: The ability to distribute your weight in a way that allows you to hold a steady position or move at will without falling.

benign paroxysmal positional vertigo (BPPV): A common balance disorder in which the canaliths inside the ear move out of place, prompting sensory hair cells to send conflicting messages about head position to the brain.

canaliths: Grains of calcium carbonate that sit on top of a layer of gel overlying sensory hair cells in the otolithic organs inside the ear. Gravity pulls on the canaliths when the head tilts. The hair cells shift in response, sending a signal to the brain describing body movements and head position.

center of gravity: The point at which your body weight is evenly distributed. Keeping your center of gravity poised over a base of support allows you to balance.

central nervous system: The brain and spinal cord. The spinal cord serves as the bridge between the brain and the body.

cerebellum: The portion of the brain, perched behind the brainstem and below the cerebral cortex, that oversees balance and movement. It synthesizes information gathered by a network of sensory nerves and issues commands.

diabetic retinopathy: An eye disorder that occurs when abnormal blood sugar levels damage small blood vessels in the retina, the light-sensitive layer at the back of the eye that captures images. Sight is blurred, and floating specks of blood can cause spots and floaters that create holes in the field of vision.

dynamic balance: The ability to anticipate and react to changes as you move.

endolymph: Fluid inside the semicircular canals of the ear.

glaucoma: A group of eye diseases that damage the optic nerve, which wires the eye to the brain. The damage usually stems from too much pressure within the eye, which kills off nerve fibers involved in vision.

labyrinthitis: A common balance disorder caused by infection or swelling in the labyrinth, the bony maze in the inner ear that plays an essential role in balance.

Ménière's disease: A common balance disorder in which fluid in the inner ear builds up until it ruptures the membranes that hold it, damaging surrounding sensory hair cells.

multiple sclerosis: An unpredictable central nervous system condition that disrupts communication between brain and body, often causing muscle weakness and interfering with balance and coordination.

osteoporosis: A condition that makes bones more porous and brittle, and thus more likely to fracture from falls.

otolithic organs: Two fluid-filled pouches inside the ear. They are paved with sensory hair cells that signal the brain about stationary head position (for example, when you are seated, leaning back, or lying down), horizontal body movement, and vertical acceleration.

Parkinson's disease: A disease that affects motor nerves throughout the body, causing tremors, rigidity of limbs and trunk, slowness of movement, and impaired balance and coordination. It is caused by the loss of brain cells that produce dopamine, a brain chemical that regulates movement, among other tasks.

peripheral nervous system: A network of nerve fibers branching out from the central nervous system throughout the rest of the body.

peripheral neuropathy: Damage to the peripheral nervous system that causes a variety of unpleasant symptoms, such as muscle weakness; shooting pains; burning; or numbness, tingling, and prickling sensations called paresthesias. Nerve fibers in the feet and legs or hands and arms often malfunction first.

proprioception: The sense of where your body is in relation to its surroundings.

proprioceptors: The position-sensing nerves responsible for proprioception, which are found in muscles, tendons, joints, and the inner ear.

semicircular canals: A trio of loops in the vestibular system inside the ear. Positioned at angles to one another, the loops are paved with sensory hair cells. The movement of fluid inside the loops causes the hair cells to tilt, setting off signals to the brain describing the position and movements of the head.

static balance: The ability to control postural sway while standing still.

vertigo: The sensation that you or the room are spinning.

vestibular disorders: A condition that affects the vestibular system, sparking trouble with balance, dizziness, and vertigo. Ear infections, head injuries, or problems with blood circulation may cause vestibular disorders.

vestibular system: A section of the inner ear that contains several structures essential to balance, including the labyrinth and the three semicircular canals.